HOLISTIC HEALTH AND WELLNESS

"The Holistic Health Guide to Wellness and Balance"

GAMALIEL O. MUDY

TABLE OF CONTENTS

PREFACE

In this enlightening journey through the pages of "Holistic Wellness," readers are transported into a world of comprehensive well-being. The book opens with an exploration of holistic health, delving into the interconnectedness of mind, body, and spirit. From the inception, the author intricately weaves together the ancient wisdom of Eastern philosophies with modern scientific understanding, laying the foundation for a holistic approach to wellness.

As the narrative unfolds, the reader is guided through the fundamentals of holistic living, embracing nutrition, exercise, and mental well-being as essential components. The book adeptly navigates through dietary principles, emphasizing the significance of whole foods, mindful eating, and the symbiotic relationship between nutrition and vitality.

Physical health takes center stage, with chapters dedicated to diverse exercise modalities, from yoga and tai chi to strength training and cardiovascular activities. The reader is not only educated on the importance of movement but also empowered to tailor a fitness routine that aligns with individual needs and preferences.

The exploration of mental well-being is a poignant highlight, offering practical strategies for stress management, mindfulness, and cultivating a positive mindset. The author seamlessly integrates practices like meditation and deep breathing, encouraging readers to foster mental resilience in the face of life's challenges.

Holistic Harmony doesn't merely stop at the individual level; it extends its reach to environmental and social dimensions. Chapters unfold with insights on sustainable living, the impact of community connections on well-being, and the reciprocal relationship between individuals and their surroundings.

The journey through the book culminates in a holistic perspective on preventive healthcare, empowering readers to take proactive measures in safeguarding their well-being. The author concludes by emphasizing the ongoing nature of the holistic wellness journey, encouraging a lifelong commitment to self-discovery and personal growth.

In "Holistic Harmony: Nurturing Wellness," readers are not only equipped with knowledge but inspired to embark on a transformative journey towards a harmonious and balanced life. This comprehensive guide serves as a beacon, illuminating the path to holistic health and wellness from its inception to an ever-evolving, enriched state of being.

CHAPTER ONE:

The Foundations of Holistic Living

Holistic living is an approach to life that emphasizes the interconnectedness of mind, body, spirit, and environment. It is a conscious and mindful way of being that seeks to create balance, harmony, and overall well-being. The foundations of holistic living encompass various aspects of our lives, encouraging a holistic mindset that extends beyond just physical health. Let's explore the key pillars that form the bedrock of holistic living.

1. Mindful Awareness:

At the core of holistic living is the cultivation of mindful awareness. This involves being present in the moment, fully engaged in your thoughts, emotions, and actions. Mindfulness practices, such as meditation and deep breathing, are powerful tools that help develop this foundational aspect, fostering mental clarity and emotional resilience.

2. Nutrient-Rich Nutrition:

Holistic living places a strong emphasis on nourishing the body through nutrient-dense, whole foods. A balanced and varied diet that includes a rainbow of fruits, vegetables, lean proteins, and whole grains supports physical health, provides sustained energy, and contributes to overall vitality.

3. Physical Well-Being:

Regular physical activity is integral to holistic living. It goes beyond structured exercise routines to encompass activities that bring joy and promote flexibility, strength, and cardiovascular health. Whether it's yoga, hiking, or dancing, finding movement that aligns with your body's needs is key to holistic well-being.

4. Emotional Wellness:

Emotional health is a cornerstone of holistic living. This involves acknowledging and processing emotions in a healthy way, cultivating positive relationships, and setting boundaries. Practices like journaling, therapy, or engaging in activities that bring joy contribute to emotional balance.

5. Spiritual Connection:

Holistic living recognizes the importance of nurturing the spirit. This doesn't necessarily mean adhering to a specific religious practice but rather connecting with something greater than oneself – whether it's nature, a higher power, or a sense of purpose. Spiritual practices, meditation, or spending time in nature can deepen this connection.

6. Environmental Consciousness:

Understanding the impact our choices have on the environment is a vital aspect of holistic living. From sustainable living practices to conscious consumerism, being environmentally aware aligns with the interconnectedness of all living things.

7. Lifelong Learning:

Holistic living thrives on a commitment to continuous learning and personal growth. This can take various forms, from acquiring new skills to exploring different perspectives. Engaging in activities that stimulate the mind and expand knowledge contributes to a holistic and fulfilling life.

In essence, the foundations of holistic living go beyond isolated lifestyle choices; they form an integrated approach to life that embraces the complexity of our existence. By nurturing these key pillars – mindful awareness, nutrient-rich nutrition, physical well-being, emotional wellness, spiritual connection, environmental consciousness, and lifelong learning – individuals can cultivate a harmonious and fulfilling life that resonates on multiple levels.

Exploring the holistic approach to health

Embarking on a journey towards holistic health is an odyssey that extends far beyond the conventional realms of physical well-being. It transcends the mere absence of illness and embraces a comprehensive, integrative approach that nurtures the body, mind, and spirit. This holistic paradigm recognizes the intricate interconnectedness of various aspects of our lives and acknowledges that optimal health arises from a harmonious balance between these dimensions.

Physical Health:

At the core of holistic health lies a profound focus on physical vitality. This encompasses not only the absence of disease but the proactive pursuit of wellness. Nutrition, exercise, and restorative sleep form the pillars of this foundation. Whole, nutrient-dense foods nourish the body, providing the essential building blocks for optimal functioning. Regular exercise, tailored to individual needs and preferences, not only enhances physical fitness but also contributes to mental and emotional well-being. Adequate and restful sleep, often overlooked in our fast-paced world, is recognized as a crucial component for overall health restoration.

Mental and Emotional Well-Being:

The holistic approach extends its reach to the intricacies of mental and emotional health. Stress, anxiety, and other emotional challenges are acknowledged as influential factors impacting physical health.

Mindfulness practices, meditation, and stress-reducing techniques are integrated into the holistic framework to foster emotional resilience. This comprehensive perspective recognizes the profound link between a calm, focused mind and the overall well-being of an individual.

Social and Environmental Considerations:

Holistic health doesn't exist in isolation; it's deeply entwined with the broader social and environmental context. Relationships, community engagement, and a sense of purpose contribute significantly to our well-being. The quality of our social connections and our connection to the environment play pivotal roles in the holistic model. Cultivating positive relationships, fostering a sense of community, and fostering an eco-conscious lifestyle are integral components.

Spiritual Wellness:

Recognizing the spiritual dimension is another cornerstone of holistic health. This doesn't necessarily imply a specific religious affiliation but rather an exploration of one's purpose, values, and connection to something greater than oneself. Practices such as meditation, prayer, or introspective activities form part of the holistic toolkit to nurture the spirit.

Personal Growth and Fulfillment:

The holistic approach encourages continual personal growth and the pursuit of fulfillment. This involves setting and striving for meaningful goals, embracing lifelong learning, and cultivating a mindset of gratitude. The fulfillment derived from aligning one's life with personal values and passions contributes significantly to overall well-being.

In essence, the holistic approach to health is a comprehensive and dynamic framework that acknowledges the intricate dance between the physical, mental, emotional, social, environmental, and spiritual aspects of our lives. It invites us to embark on a journey of self-discovery and self-care, fostering a harmonious balance that propels us towards a state of flourishing vitality and enduring well-being. As we navigate this holistic terrain, we uncover the interconnected threads that weave together the rich tapestry of our health and ultimately shape the quality of our lives.

Understanding the interconnectedness of mind, body, and spirit

Understanding the interconnectedness of mind, body, and spirit is a profound exploration into the holistic nature of human existence. In this intricate dance of elements, each facet - mind, body, and spirit - is not an isolated entity but rather a vital thread woven into the intricate fabric of our being.

The mind, often considered the epicenter of consciousness, is a dynamic landscape where thoughts, emotions, and perceptions converge. It's the reservoir of our intellect, creativity, and self-awareness. The mind shapes our beliefs, influences our attitudes, and navigates the complex terrain of our experiences. Its interconnectedness with the body and spirit is palpable, as thoughts can influence physical health and spiritual well-being.

The body, our tangible and resilient vessel, is an embodiment of our existence. Its health, vitality, and functionality are intimately linked to the mind and spirit. The mind-body connection is evident in the impact of thoughts and emotions on physical health. Stress, for instance, can manifest as physical ailments, highlighting the intricate interplay between mental well-being and bodily health.

The spirit, often considered the essence of our being, transcends the tangible boundaries of the mind and body. It's the source of our inner strength, resilience, and connection to something greater than ourselves. The spiritual dimension adds depth and meaning to our lives, influencing our values, purpose, and sense of interconnectedness with the world around us.

This interconnectedness is not a one-way street but a dynamic exchange. A healthy mind contributes to physical well-being, just as physical vitality can enhance mental clarity. Meanwhile, a nurtured spirit can infuse both mind and body with a sense of purpose and resilience. It's a symbiotic relationship where the well-being of one element ripples through and enriches the others.

Recognizing and nurturing this interconnectedness is key to holistic well-being. Practices such as mindfulness, meditation, and holistic health approaches acknowledge the profound interplay between mind, body, and spirit. By cultivating awareness and harmony across these dimensions, individuals can embark on a journey towards a more balanced, fulfilling, and integrated existence.

In essence, understanding the interconnectedness of mind, body, and spirit is an invitation to explore the richness of our humanity. It encourages a holistic approach to health and well-being, recognizing that true vitality arises not from isolating these elements but from embracing the synergy that emerges when mind, body, and spirit dance in harmony.

Embracing Holistic Health and Wellness.

In a fast-paced world, where the demands of modern life often take precedence, the pursuit of holistic health and wellness stands out as a transformative journey towards a more balanced and fulfilling existence. Holistic health extends beyond the mere absence of illness; it encompasses a profound sense of well-being that integrates the physical, mental, emotional, and spiritual aspects of an individual's life.

Physical Well-Being:

At the core of holistic health lies the recognition that the body is a complex and interconnected system. Prioritizing physical health involves nourishing the body with wholesome nutrition, engaging in regular exercise, and ensuring adequate rest and recovery. This holistic approach acknowledges that physical well-being is not just about the absence of disease but about optimizing the body's potential for vitality and resilience.

Mental and Emotional Harmony:

Holistic health emphasizes the inseparable connection between mental and physical well-being. Practices such as mindfulness, meditation, and stress management play a crucial role in cultivating mental clarity and emotional balance. Recognizing and addressing the sources of stress, anxiety, and emotional turmoil contributes to a more harmonious internal landscape, fostering a sense of peace and stability.

Nutritional Wisdom:

Nutrition is a cornerstone of holistic health, emphasizing the importance of mindful and nourishing food choices. Beyond mere sustenance, holistic nutrition recognizes food as medicine, acknowledging its power to heal and support the body. This approach encourages a diverse, plant-based diet rich in nutrients, aligning with the body's natural processes for optimal digestion, absorption, and overall well-being.

Spiritual Connection:

Holistic health recognizes the spiritual dimension as an integral part of a person's overall wellness. This doesn't necessarily align with a specific religious belief but rather encourages individuals to explore and nurture a sense of purpose, meaning, and connection to something greater than themselves. Spiritual practices, whether through meditation, prayer, or nature connection, contribute to a deeper understanding of one's existence and purpose.

Lifestyle Choices and Environmental Harmony:

A holistic approach extends to lifestyle choices and the environment in which one lives. Sustainable and conscious living aligns with holistic health principles, recognizing the impact of personal choices on both individual well-being and the health of the planet. This involves making choices that support both personal health and the health of the broader community and ecosystem.

Interpersonal Relationships:

Holistic health emphasizes the significance of positive and nurturing relationships. Healthy connections with family, friends, and the community contribute significantly to emotional well-being. Cultivating meaningful relationships fosters a sense of support, belonging, and interconnectedness, promoting overall mental and emotional health.

Mind-Body Practices:

Incorporating mind-body practices such as yoga, tai chi, or qigong into daily routines enhances the mind-body connection. These practices not only promote physical flexibility and strength but also cultivate mindfulness, relaxation, and a deeper understanding of the body's signals.

Embracing holistic health and wellness is an ongoing, dynamic process that invites individuals to become active participants in their own well-being. It's about recognizing the intricate interplay of various elements that contribute to a fulfilling and balanced life.

By integrating physical, mental, emotional, and spiritual aspects, holistic health offers a comprehensive approach to not just surviving but thriving in the modern world. As you embark on this journey, may you find empowerment, joy, and a renewed sense of vitality.

Emphasizing the importance of a holistic foundation for overall well-being

In the pursuit of a fulfilling and meaningful life, it's crucial to recognize the integral role a holistic foundation plays in shaping our overall well-being. Holistic well-being encompasses not just physical health but extends to mental, emotional, social, and even spiritual aspects of our lives. It is the interconnectedness of these dimensions that forms the essence of a comprehensive approach to wellness.

At the core of holistic well-being is the acknowledgment that our physical health is intricately linked to our mental and emotional states. When we prioritize activities that nurture our bodies, such as regular exercise, a balanced diet, and sufficient rest, we not only enhance our physical vitality but also lay the groundwork for improved mental clarity and emotional resilience. The mind and body are not isolated entities; they function harmoniously, and their synergy is the cornerstone of a holistic foundation.

Mental well-being, often underestimated, holds profound significance in our overall health. Stress, anxiety, and other mental health challenges can have tangible effects on our physical health. Cultivating practices like mindfulness, meditation, or engaging in activities that bring joy and purpose can significantly contribute to mental resilience. These practices not only foster a positive mindset but also serve as effective tools in managing life's inevitable challenges.

Emotional well-being, another integral component of the holistic framework, involves understanding, expressing, and navigating our emotions in a healthy way. Building strong emotional intelligence allows us to form meaningful connections with others and ourselves. Social interactions, relationships, and a sense of community play pivotal roles in shaping emotional well-being. Nurturing healthy relationships, practicing empathy, and fostering social connections contribute profoundly to our overall happiness.

Moreover, the spiritual dimension adds depth to our holistic foundation. This doesn't necessarily refer to religious beliefs but encompasses a sense of purpose, meaning, and connection to something greater than ourselves. It involves aligning our actions with our values, finding a sense of purpose, and fostering inner peace. Individuals who cultivate spiritual well-being often report a greater sense of fulfillment and resilience in the face of life's challenges.

In essence, the importance of a holistic foundation for overall well-being lies in recognizing that we are complex beings with interconnected facets. Neglecting one aspect can have a ripple effect on others. By embracing a holistic approach, we empower ourselves to lead more fulfilling lives, where physical health, mental clarity, emotional resilience, social connections, and a sense of purpose converge to create a harmonious and flourishing existence. It's an invitation to embark on a journey towards a more balanced and meaningful life—one where each dimension of our well-being contributes to the vibrant tapestry of our holistic health.

In the pursuit of a fulfilling and balanced life, establishing a holistic foundation is paramount to achieving overall well-being. Holistic well-being transcends the narrow focus on physical health and extends its embrace to mental, emotional, social, and even spiritual dimensions. This comprehensive approach recognizes the interconnectedness of various aspects of our lives, fostering a state of equilibrium that goes beyond mere absence of illness. Let's delve into the multifaceted significance of a holistic foundation for a flourishing and vibrant existence.

Physical Well-being:

A robust foundation begins with physical health. Regular exercise, balanced nutrition, and sufficient rest are the cornerstones that energize our bodies and fortify our immune systems. By nurturing our physical well-being, we create a resilient base that allows us to tackle life's challenges with vitality and vigor.

Mental and Emotional Harmony:

True well-being extends into the realms of mental and emotional health. Cultivating mindfulness, managing stress, and fostering emotional intelligence are vital components of a holistic foundation. When we prioritize our mental and emotional well-being, we enhance our ability to cope with adversity, make sound decisions, and forge meaningful connections with others.

Social Connections:

Human beings are inherently social creatures, and our well-being is profoundly influenced by the quality of our relationships. A holistic foundation emphasizes the importance of nurturing social connections, fostering a sense of belonging, and cultivating healthy communication. Meaningful relationships contribute to emotional support, shared experiences, and a profound sense of purpose.

Professional and Financial Wellness:

Career satisfaction and financial stability contribute significantly to our overall well-being. A holistic approach involves aligning our professional endeavors with our values and passions, promoting a sense of purpose and fulfillment. Concurrently, prudent financial management creates a stable platform, alleviating stress and ensuring our ability to meet our basic needs and pursue our aspirations.

Spiritual Fulfillment:

Holistic well-being also encompasses spiritual dimensions. This doesn't necessarily imply adherence to a specific religious doctrine but rather finding a sense of purpose, connection, and transcendence. Exploring one's values, engaging in introspection, and connecting with a higher purpose contribute to a profound sense of spiritual fulfillment.

Balance and Equilibrium:

At the heart of a holistic foundation lies the pursuit of balance. Balancing the various facets of our lives prevents the undue dominance of one aspect at the expense of others. It involves setting boundaries, prioritizing self-care, and recognizing that true well-being arises from the harmonious integration of diverse elements.

In essence, emphasizing the importance of a holistic foundation for overall well-being is an acknowledgment that we are intricate beings with interconnected dimensions. By nurturing each aspect—physical, mental, emotional, social, professional, financial, and spiritual—we pave the way for a life that is not only healthy but also fulfilling and resilient. It's an investment in ourselves that pays dividends in the form of sustained joy, purpose, and a profound sense of contentment.

CHAPTER TWO:

Nourishing Your Body with Whole Foods

In an era dominated by processed and convenience foods, the concept of nourishing your body with whole foods has emerged as a beacon of health and vitality. Whole foods, in their unprocessed, natural state, provide a plethora of nutrients that promote overall well-being, enhance energy levels, and contribute to a resilient immune system. In this comprehensive guide, we will explore the multifaceted benefits of embracing a diet rich in whole foods, along with practical tips for incorporating them into your daily life.

Understanding Whole Foods:
Whole foods are minimally processed and free from additives, preserving their nutritional

integrity. These include fruits, vegetables, whole grains, lean proteins, nuts, and seeds. Unlike their processed counterparts, whole foods retain their original nutrients, fiber, and phytochemicals, offering a holistic approach to nutrition.

The Nutritional Powerhouse:

Whole foods are nature's nutritional powerhouse, providing a diverse array of essential vitamins, minerals, antioxidants, and fiber. These nutrients work synergistically to support optimal health, from bolstering the immune system to promoting cardiovascular well-being and maintaining healthy skin and hair.

Benefits for Weight Management:

Whole foods, with their high fiber content, contribute to a feeling of fullness, aiding in weight management. Unlike processed foods laden with empty calories, whole foods provide sustained energy, reducing the likelihood of overeating and supporting healthy weight goals.

Balancing Blood Sugar Levels:
A diet based on whole foods helps stabilize blood sugar levels. The gradual release of carbohydrates from whole grains and the fiber content of fruits and vegetables prevent spikes and crashes in blood sugar, reducing the risk of type 2 diabetes and promoting sustained energy throughout the day.

Supporting Digestive Health:
Whole foods, especially those high in fiber, promote digestive health by preventing constipation and supporting a diverse and thriving gut microbiome. A healthy gut is

linked to improved immunity, mood regulation, and even cognitive function.

Practical Tips for Incorporation:

Diversify Your Plate: Aim for a colorful array of fruits and vegetables to ensure a broad spectrum of nutrients.

1. **Choose Whole Grains**: Opt for whole grains like quinoa, brown rice, and oats over refined grains for enhanced fiber and nutrient content.
2. Include Lean Proteins: Incorporate lean proteins such as poultry, fish, legumes, and tofu for sustained energy and muscle health.
3. **Snack Smartly**: Choose whole food snacks like fresh fruits, nuts, and yogurt over processed snacks for sustained energy.

Nourishing your body with whole foods is a fundamental step towards achieving optimal health and vitality. By embracing the inherent goodness of unprocessed, natural foods, you provide your body with the tools it needs to thrive. The benefits extend beyond physical well-being to encompass mental clarity, emotional balance, and a heightened overall quality of life. So, embark on this journey of wholesome nutrition, savor the richness of whole foods, and witness the transformative power they bring to every aspect of your well-being.

The Role of Nutrition in holistic health

In the intricate tapestry of holistic health, nutrition emerges as a cornerstone, weaving its threads through the interconnected realms of the mind, body, and soul. This comprehensive approach transcends mere dietary choices; it encapsulates a lifestyle that recognizes the profound impact of nutrition on our overall well-being.

1. Physical Well-Being:

Nutrition serves as the building blocks for physical health. A well-balanced and nutrient-rich diet provides the body with the essential elements it needs to function optimally. From vitamins and minerals to proteins and carbohydrates, each component plays a crucial role in maintaining bodily functions, supporting metabolism, and fortifying the immune system. Whole, unprocessed foods become the fuel that powers the intricate machinery of our bodies. Antioxidants present in fruits and vegetables combat oxidative stress, reducing inflammation and contributing to the prevention of chronic diseases. Nutrient-dense foods, such as lean proteins and whole grains, become allies in maintaining healthy weight, stabilizing blood sugar levels, and promoting cardiovascular health.

2. Mental Clarity and Cognitive Function:

The intimate connection between nutrition and mental well-being is undeniable. The brain, an organ of immense complexity, relies on a steady supply of nutrients for optimal function. Omega-3 fatty acids, found in abundance in fatty fish and certain seeds, are known to support cognitive function and play a role in mental health.Additionally, the gut-brain axis highlights the relationship between the digestive system and mental health. A diet rich in probiotics and prebiotics fosters a healthy gut microbiome, influencing neurotransmitter production and positively impacting mood and cognitive function.

3. Emotional Balance:

Nutrition is intricately linked to emotional health, with certain foods influencing the production of neurotransmitters that regulate mood. Serotonin, often referred to as the "feel-good" neurotransmitter, is influenced by the amino acid tryptophan found in foods like turkey, nuts, and seeds. Consuming a balanced diet that supports the production of such neurotransmitters contributes to emotional stability and resilience.

4. Spiritual Nourishment:

Holistic health extends beyond the physical and mental realms, embracing the spiritual dimension of our existence. Nutrition, in this context, becomes a means of spiritual nourishment, fostering a connection to the environment, the community, and the self. Mindful eating practices, such as savoring each bite and expressing gratitude for the sustenance received, elevate the act of nourishment to a spiritual experience.

5. Disease Prevention and Longevity:

A nutrient-rich diet is a powerful tool in the prevention of diseases, promoting longevity and vitality. The anti-inflammatory properties of certain foods, such as turmeric and berries, contribute to the prevention of chronic conditions. Antioxidant-rich foods neutralize free radicals, reducing the risk of cellular damage and supporting overall health.

In conclusion, the role of nutrition in holistic health is multifaceted, encompassing physical, mental, emotional, and spiritual well-being. A conscious and balanced approach to food choices becomes a transformative journey towards optimal health, aligning the mind, body, and soul in harmony. Embracing the profound impact of nutrition is not just a dietary choice; it is a commitment to a life of vitality, resilience, and holistic wellness.

Exploring whole foods, mindful eating, and nutrition's impact on well-being

In our fast-paced world, where convenience often takes precedence over consciousness, the relationship between our dietary choices and overall well-being becomes increasingly paramount. This exploration delves into the profound intersection of whole foods, mindful eating, and the pivotal role nutrition plays in nurturing not just our bodies, but our holistic sense of health and vitality.

Understanding Whole Foods:

Whole foods refer to natural, unprocessed, and minimally refined ingredients that retain their nutritional integrity. Fruits, vegetables, whole grains, nuts, seeds, and lean proteins exemplify the essence of whole foods. The key lies in embracing these nutrient-dense options in their unadulterated state, harnessing the benefits of a myriad of vitamins, minerals, and antioxidants that contribute to our well-being.

Whole foods offer a symphony of nutrients, each playing a unique role in supporting bodily functions. From the fiber in fruits and vegetables promoting digestive health to the omega-3 fatty acids in certain nuts and fish fostering cardiovascular well-being, the holistic approach of whole foods nourishes us on a cellular level.

The Art of Mindful Eating:

Mindful eating transcends the act of consumption; it's a conscious and intentional approach to nourishing our bodies. In a world filled with distractions, adopting mindfulness during meals becomes a transformative practice. This involves savoring each bite, appreciating the flavors, textures, and aromas, and listening to our body's hunger and fullness cues.

By fostering a mindful eating practice, we cultivate a deeper connection with our food and, subsequently, our bodies. This approach encourages us to eat with intention, addressing not only the nutritional needs but also the emotional and psychological aspects of our relationship with food.

Nutrition's Impact on Well-being:

The significance of nutrition in shaping our well-being cannot be overstated. Beyond the immediate physical effects, our dietary choices influence mental clarity, emotional stability, and long-term health outcomes.

Adequate nutrition supports optimal brain function, contributes to mood regulation, and plays a pivotal role in preventing chronic diseases.

Balanced nutrition involves a harmonious blend of macronutrients (carbohydrates, proteins, and fats) and micronutrients (vitamins and minerals). Striking this balance ensures our bodies receive the fuel necessary for energy, growth, and repair. It also strengthens our immune system, enhances cognitive function, and aids in maintaining a healthy weight.

Practical Steps Towards Holistic Well-being:

1. **Embrace a Plant Based Focus:** Prioritize colorful fruits and vegetables, whole grains, and plant-based proteins for a diverse range of nutrients.

2. **Practice Mindful Eating Rituals:** Create a conducive environment for meals, minimize distractions, and savor each bite with gratitude and awareness.

3. **Educate Yourself:** Stay informed about the nutritional content of the foods you consume, and make informed choices that align with your health goals.

4. **Hydrate Adequately:** Water is an essential component of well-being. Ensure you stay adequately hydrated to support bodily functions.

5. **Cultivate Balance, Not Deprivation:** Strive for a balanced diet that includes a variety of foods. Allow yourself occasional treats, fostering a

sustainable and enjoyable approach to nutrition.

The synergy of whole foods, mindful eating, and nutrition offers a holistic pathway to well-being. By nurturing our bodies with intention and fueling them with the richness of nature's bounty, we lay the foundation for a vibrant and fulfilling life. This journey is not just about what we eat but how we approach nourishment – a celebration of the intricate dance between mindful choices and the profound impact they have on our physical, mental, and emotional well-being.

Encouraging a balanced, whole-foods-based diet for optimal health

In a world where dietary trends often come and go, the timeless wisdom of encouraging a balanced, whole-foods-based diet stands as a beacon for optimal health. This approach to nourishment goes beyond mere calorie counting; it's a holistic philosophy that views food as more than just sustenance but as a powerful contributor to overall well-being.

Understanding Whole Foods:

At the core of this dietary philosophy is a focus on whole foods – those that are as close to their natural state as possible. Think vibrant fruits, colorful vegetables, lean proteins, whole grains, and nuts. These foods are nutrient-dense, providing a spectrum of vitamins, minerals, antioxidants, and fiber crucial for the body's optimal functioning.

Balancing Macronutrients:

A balanced diet involves the right proportion of macronutrients – proteins, fats, and carbohydrates. Proteins, found in sources like lean meats, beans, and dairy, are essential for muscle repair and overall cellular function. Healthy fats, from sources like avocados and nuts, support brain health and aid in nutrient absorption. Complex carbohydrates, abundant in whole grains and vegetables, offer sustained energy and essential fiber for digestive health.

The Power of Nutrient Density:

Whole foods are inherently nutrient-dense, meaning they provide a high concentration of essential nutrients relative to their calorie content. This density ensures that each bite contributes not only to satiety but also to the body's nutritional needs, fostering optimal health from the inside out.

Fostering Digestive Wellness:

The fiber present in whole foods is a cornerstone of digestive health. It promotes regular bowel movements, helps maintain a healthy weight, and supports the growth of beneficial gut bacteria. A well-functioning digestive system is key to nutrient absorption and the elimination of waste, contributing to overall vitality.

Mindful Eating Practices:

Encouraging a whole-foods-based diet goes hand-in-hand with adopting mindful eating practices. This involves savoring each bite, paying attention to hunger and fullness cues, and cultivating a deeper connection with the food on one's plate. By fostering a mindful relationship with food, individuals can enhance their appreciation for the nourishing qualities of whole foods.

Disease Prevention and Longevity:

Scientific studies consistently highlight the role of a balanced, whole-foods-based diet in preventing chronic diseases such as heart disease, diabetes, and certain cancers. The rich array of antioxidants found in fruits and vegetables, for example, helps combat oxidative stress and inflammation, contributing to a lower risk of these diseases. Longevity, too, is often associated with diets rich in whole, nutrient-dense foods.

Practical Tips for Implementation:

Making the shift toward a whole-foods-based diet can be approached gradually. Begin by incorporating more colorful fruits and vegetables into meals, opting for whole grains instead of refined ones, and choosing lean protein sources. Experiment with herbs and spices to enhance flavor without relying on excessive salt or sugar. Gradually reducing processed foods and sugar intake can also contribute to a healthier dietary pattern.

In conclusion, encouraging a balanced, whole-foods-based diet is a timeless prescription for optimal health. It's a celebration of the abundance nature provides, a commitment to nourishing the body with wholesome goodness, and a pathway to not only physical well-being but also to a deeper connection with the vitality of life. By embracing this holistic approach to nutrition, individuals can cultivate habits that support their health today and lay the foundation for a vibrant and resilient future.

CHAPTER THREE:

Mindfulness and Stress Management

In the hustle and bustle of our fast-paced lives, the art of mindfulness and stress management has emerged as a beacon of serenity. Mindfulness, rooted in ancient contemplative practices, is a powerful tool that transcends time, offering a profound way to navigate the challenges of our modern world.

At its core, mindfulness is a state of heightened awareness, an intentional focus on the present moment without judgment. In a society where multitasking has become a badge of honor, mindfulness invites us to savor each moment, fostering a sense of clarity and calm amid life's chaos.

Understanding Mindfulness:

Mindfulness invites us to be fully present, acknowledging our thoughts and feelings without getting entangled in them. It's not about erasing stressors but rather about changing our relationship with them. By cultivating this awareness, we can respond to stressors with intention rather than reacting impulsively.

The Stress Epidemic:

In a world marked by constant connectivity and information overload, stress has become an ever-present companion. From workplace pressures to personal challenges, stress can manifest physically and emotionally, taking a toll on our well-being. Mindfulness offers a sanctuary amidst this chaos, providing a pause button that allows us to respond to stressors with a measured and composed demeanor.

Mindfulness Practices for Stress Management:

Mindfulness is not a one-size-fits-all approach; it encompasses various practices tailored to individual preferences. Meditation, a cornerstone of mindfulness, involves focusing attention on the breath or a specific point, fostering a quiet mind. Mindful breathing, body scan meditations, and guided imagery are valuable tools in developing this mental discipline.

Additionally, mindful movement practices like yoga offer a kinesthetic approach to mindfulness, integrating breath with physical postures. Engaging in these practices regularly promotes a sense of inner balance, reducing the physiological markers of stress and enhancing overall well-being.

The Science Behind Mindfulness:

Scientific studies underscore the efficacy of mindfulness in stress reduction. Research suggests that regular mindfulness practice can alter the brain's structure, particularly in areas associated with emotional regulation and self-awareness. Furthermore, studies indicate that mindfulness can reduce the production of stress hormones, fostering a physiological state conducive to relaxation.

Integrating Mindfulness into Daily Life:

The true power of mindfulness lies in its integration into daily life. From mindful eating to incorporating moments of stillness into a hectic schedule, small but consistent practices can yield significant benefits. Mindfulness is not an escape from reality but a way to engage with it more skillfully, fostering resilience in the face of life's inevitable challenges

In the symphony of modern living, mindfulness serves as a soothing melody, offering a counterpoint to the cacophony of stress. Through intentional presence and a commitment to self-awareness, we can cultivate a resilient mindset that navigates life's complexities with grace. Mindfulness and stress management are not fleeting trends but timeless practices that empower us to live more fully and authentically in every moment. Embrace the journey inward, and let mindfulness be your guide to a more balanced and harmonious existence

CHAPTER FOUR:

The mind-body connection and its impact on health

The intricate interplay between the mind and the body is a fascinating and profound phenomenon that has captivated the attention of researchers, healthcare professionals, and individuals seeking holistic well-being. The mind-body connection goes beyond a simple acknowledgment that mental and physical health are intertwined; it delves into the complex ways in which thoughts, emotions, and physiological responses harmonize to influence overall health.

At the heart of this intricate relationship is the understanding that our thoughts and emotions can significantly impact our physical well-being. The power of the mind to shape the body's responses is evident in various aspects of health, from immune function to cardiovascular health. Studies have shown that chronic stress, often rooted in mental and emotional factors, can compromise the immune system, making the body more susceptible to illnesses. Conversely, positive emotions and a healthy mental state have been associated with improved immune function and better overall health.

One remarkable aspect of the mind-body connection is its influence on the autonomic nervous system, which regulates involuntary bodily functions such as heart rate, digestion, and respiratory rate. Stressful thoughts or emotions can trigger the sympathetic nervous system, commonly known as the "fight or flight" response, leading to increased heart rate, heightened alertness, and other physiological changes. On the other hand, relaxation techniques and positive mental states can activate the parasympathetic nervous system, promoting relaxation, improved digestion, and a sense of well-being.

Moreover, the impact of the mind on chronic conditions cannot be overstated. Conditions such as chronic pain, autoimmune disorders, and gastrointestinal issues often exhibit connections to stress, anxiety, or unresolved emotional factors. Integrative approaches that address both the physical and psychological aspects of these conditions have shown promising results in improving symptoms and enhancing overall quality of life.

The mind-body connection extends its influence to the realm of lifestyle choices. Health behaviors such as diet, exercise, and sleep are deeply intertwined with mental and emotional well-being. Stress, for example, can contribute to unhealthy eating patterns, disrupted sleep, and decreased motivation for physical activity. Recognizing and addressing the psychological components of these behaviors is crucial for establishing sustainable, health-promoting habits.

Mind-body practices have gained widespread recognition for their positive impact on overall health. Techniques such as meditation, yoga, and mindfulness are designed to foster a harmonious connection between the mind and body. These practices have been linked to stress reduction, improved emotional well-being, and even physiological benefits such as lowered blood pressure and enhanced immune function, the mind-body connection is a profound and dynamic relationship that significantly influences health outcomes. Understanding and harnessing this connection can empower individuals to take an active role in their well-being. Adopting holistic approaches that consider both mental and physical aspects of health is essential for achieving optimal wellness and fostering a balanced and harmonious relationship between the mind and the body.

At its core, the mind-body connection reflects the inseparable nature of our thoughts, emotions, and physiological responses. Consider the experience of stress – a mental state that triggers a cascade of physical reactions. When stressed, the body releases hormones like cortisol and adrenaline, leading to increased heart rate, elevated blood pressure, and even changes in digestion. This exemplifies how our mental state directly influences our bodily functions.

Positive emotions, on the other hand, can contribute to improved health. Happiness, gratitude, and contentment are linked to the release of endorphins, the body's natural feel-good chemicals. These substances not only enhance mood but also act as natural painkillers, highlighting the intricate ways in which positive mental states can positively influence physical well-being.

Conversely, chronic negative emotions or stress can contribute to various health issues. Research suggests that prolonged stress may weaken the immune system, making individuals more susceptible to illnesses.

Additionally, it can contribute to the development or exacerbation of conditions such as cardiovascular disease, digestive disorders, and even chronic pain.

The impact of the mind-body connection extends beyond the immediate physiological responses. Consider the placebo effect, where the belief in the effectiveness of a treatment influences the body's response, even if the treatment itself lacks therapeutic properties. This phenomenon underscores the role of our beliefs and perceptions in shaping our physical experiences.

Mind-body practices, such as meditation, yoga, and mindfulness, have gained popularity as holistic approaches to health. These practices emphasize the integration of mental and physical well-being, promoting relaxation, stress reduction, and enhanced self-awareness. Numerous studies suggest that incorporating such practices into one's routine can positively impact various health markers, from reducing blood pressure to improving mental clarity.

In the realm of chronic illnesses, the mind-body connection plays a crucial role. Conditions like fibromyalgia, irritable bowel syndrome (IBS), and chronic fatigue syndrome are often influenced by both psychological and physiological factors. Integrative approaches that address both the mental and physical aspects of these conditions have shown promising results in managing symptoms and improving overall quality of life.

The mind-body connection is not a one-size-fits-all concept; its manifestation varies among individuals. Factors such as genetics, upbringing, and personal experiences contribute to the complexity of this relationship. Acknowledging and understanding this connection opens doors to holistic approaches to health that consider not only physical symptoms but also the emotional and psychological aspects of well-being.

In conclusion, the mind-body connection stands as a testament to the profound unity of our mental and physical selves. Nurturing this connection through mindful practices, positive mental states, and a holistic approach to health can pave the way for a more vibrant and balanced life. As we continue to unravel the mysteries of this intricate relationship, we gain insights that empower us to take charge of our well-being in ways that extend beyond the confines of the physical body.

Techniques for mindfulness, stress reduction, and mental well-being
In the fast-paced world we live in, characterized by constant connectivity and information overload, maintaining mental well-being is more crucial than ever. Techniques for mindfulness and stress reduction provide a sanctuary amidst the chaos, offering a path towards tranquility and balance. In this exploration, we delve into a variety of practices that go beyond mere relaxation – they cultivate a profound sense of mindfulness and contribute to overall mental well-being.

Mindfulness Meditation:

At the core of mindfulness techniques lies meditation. Mindfulness meditation encourages individuals to focus on the present moment, acknowledging thoughts without judgment. By cultivating this awareness, individuals can reduce stress and gain a deeper understanding of their emotions and reactions.

Deep Breathing Exercises:

Conscious and deep breathing serves as an immediate antidote to stress. Techniques such as diaphragmatic breathing or the 4-7-8 technique promote relaxation by calming the nervous system or paced breathing help activate the body's relaxation response, calming the nervous system and promoting mental and emotional clarity.

Progressive Muscle Relaxation:

This technique involves systematically tensing and then relaxing different muscle groups, promoting physical and mental relaxation. Progressive muscle relaxation is particularly effective in alleviating tension and stress stored in the body.

Body Scan Meditation:

A body scan involves directing focused attention to different parts of the body, observing sensations without judgment. This practice enhances self-awareness and promotes a connection between the mind and body, aiding in stress reduction.

Visualization and Guided Imagery:

Immersing oneself in positive and calming mental images can significantly reduce stress. Guided imagery, led by soothing narration or self-created visualizations, transports individuals to serene mental landscapes, fostering relaxation and a break from daily stressors.

Yoga for Mind-Body Harmony:

Yoga combines physical postures, breath control, and meditation. Its holistic approach not only enhances physical flexibility but also promotes mental well-being. Regular yoga practice has been linked to reduced stress, anxiety, and improved overall mood.

Journaling for Emotional Release:

Putting pen to paper offers a tangible outlet for emotions. Journaling allows individuals to explore their thoughts, identify patterns, and release pent-up emotions. It's a therapeutic practice that promotes self-reflection and emotional well-being.

Mindful Walking:

The simple act of walking can transform into a mindfulness practice. Engaging in mindful walking involves paying attention to each step, the sensation of movement, and the connection with the environment. This technique fosters a sense of grounding and presence, offering a reprieve from the chaos of the mind.

Mindful Eating Practices:

Mindful eating involves savoring each bite, paying attention to flavors, textures, and the overall eating experience. This practice not only fosters a healthier relationship with food but also encourages a mindful approach to daily activities.

Nature Connection and Grounding Techniques:

Spending time in nature or incorporating grounding techniques, like walking barefoot on grass, can have a profound impact on mental well-being. The simplicity of connecting with the natural world brings a sense of calm and perspective.

Gratitude Practices:

Cultivating a mindset of gratitude involves acknowledging and appreciating the positive aspects of life. Regularly expressing gratitude, whether through journaling or verbal affirmations, can shift focus towards positivity, reducing stress and enhancing overall mental well-being.

Yoga and Tai Chi:

Mindful movement practices like yoga and Tai Chi combine physical postures with breath awareness. These ancient disciplines not only promote flexibility and strength but also contribute significantly to mental well-being by encouraging a harmonious connection between body and mind.

In integrating these techniques into our lives, we embark on a journey towards greater mindfulness, reduced stress, and enhanced mental well-being. Each approach offers a unique avenue for self-discovery and personal growth. As we embrace these practices, we open doors to a more tranquil and fulfilling existence in our ever-evolving quest for a balanced and healthy mind.

Incorporating these mindfulness and stress reduction techniques into daily life offers a holistic approach to mental well-being. The key lies in consistency and the cultivation of self-awareness, creating a foundation for resilience and balance in the face of life's challenges

Emphasizing the transformative power of mindfulness in holistic health

In the bustling pace of modern life, where stress and demands often take center stage, the transformative power of mindfulness emerges as a beacon of hope, offering a profound pathway to holistic health. Beyond a fleeting buzzword, mindfulness is a way of life, a practice that extends far beyond the realms of stress reduction. It's a transformative force that permeates every facet of our existence, from physical well-being to mental resilience, fostering a harmonious synergy between mind, body, and spirit.

At its core, mindfulness is about presence – a conscious and intentional awareness of the present moment without judgment. In the context of holistic health, this practice becomes a cornerstone, allowing individuals to reconnect with their inner selves and the world around them. The ripple effects of mindfulness extend far beyond the immediate calm it brings; it acts as a catalyst for a profound shift in perspective and approach to life.

In terms of mental health, mindfulness serves as a formidable ally against the chaos of the mind. It invites individuals to observe their thoughts and emotions with a non-judgmental lens, creating a space for self-reflection and understanding. This heightened awareness is a transformative journey inward, uncovering patterns of thinking and behaviors that may hinder optimal well-being.

Moreover, the impact of mindfulness radiates into the physical realm, influencing the body's response to stress and contributing to overall vitality. Mindful practices such as deep breathing, meditation, and gentle movement foster a holistic integration of mind and body, promoting relaxation, reducing inflammation, and even influencing the expression of certain genes associated with health.

Holistic health is not just about the absence of illness but the presence of vitality and flourishing in every aspect of life. Mindfulness becomes the bridge connecting the dots of mental, emotional, and physical well-being. It invites individuals to savor the richness of each moment, fostering gratitude and resilience even in the face of challenges.

Furthermore, the transformative power of mindfulness extends into the realm of interpersonal relationships. As individuals become more attuned to their own thoughts and emotions, they naturally develop a heightened sense of empathy and compassion for others. Mindfulness cultivates deep connections, fostering a sense of community and shared humanity that contributes to emotional well-being.

In essence, embracing mindfulness as a core element of holistic health is an investment in one's own flourishing. It transcends a mere stress management tool and becomes a way of living consciously and authentically. The journey of mindfulness is a continuous exploration, an unwavering commitment to self-discovery, and a realization that true well-being is a tapestry woven with threads of presence, compassion, and an abiding connection to the beauty of life in all its dimensions.

CHAPTER FIVE:

Holistic Fitness and Exercise

Holistic fitness and exercise represent a comprehensive approach to well-being, acknowledging that true health extends beyond mere physical strength to encompass mental, emotional, and spiritual aspects. In the pursuit of holistic fitness, individuals seek a balanced and integrated lifestyle that nurtures every facet of their being.

Understanding Holistic Fitness:

Holistic fitness is rooted in the understanding that the body, mind, and spirit are interconnected, influencing each other profoundly. It goes beyond the conventional notion of exercise solely for physical benefits and delves into practices that enhance overall vitality and longevity.

Physical Exercise as a Pillar:

While physical exercise is a central component, holistic fitness broadens the scope beyond traditional workouts. It encourages diverse activities such as yoga, tai chi, and dance, recognizing that movement can be both therapeutic and enjoyable. This inclusive approach fosters adaptability, ensuring that individuals can tailor their fitness routines to suit their preferences and needs.

Mind-Body Connection:

A key tenet of holistic fitness is the acknowledgment of the mind-body connection. Practices like mindfulness meditation and breathwork are integrated into routines, promoting mental clarity, stress reduction, and emotional well-being. This holistic approach recognizes that mental health is as crucial as physical fitness for overall vitality.

Nutrition as Nourishment:

Holistic fitness places a strong emphasis on nutrition as a form of self-care. It goes beyond calorie counting, encouraging mindful eating and the consumption of whole, nutrient-dense foods. This approach recognizes that food is not just fuel but a vital source of energy that affects every aspect of one's well-being.

Rest and Recovery:

Holistic fitness recognizes the importance of rest and recovery in the overall health equation. Quality sleep, relaxation techniques, and adequate downtime are integrated into the fitness philosophy, understanding that the body requires time to rejuvenate and repair.

Embracing Holistic Practices:

Holistic fitness extends beyond the gym or yoga studio. It encompasses lifestyle choices that contribute to a holistic approach to health, such as fostering positive relationships, cultivating a sense of purpose, and engaging in activities that bring joy and fulfillment.

Spiritual Well-being:

For many practitioners of holistic fitness, spiritual well-being is a crucial component. This doesn't necessarily imply adherence to a specific religion but rather a connection to a higher purpose, whether through nature, mindfulness practices, or personal philosophy.

Personalization and Adaptability:

What sets holistic fitness apart is its recognition that there is no one-size-fits-all approach. It encourages individuals to listen to their bodies, adapt their routines as needed, and personalize their fitness journeys based on their unique circumstances and goals.

The Holistic Fitness Journey:

Embarking on a holistic fitness journey is an invitation to explore the interconnectedness of body, mind, and spirit. It's a commitment to self-discovery, growth, and a harmonious approach to well-being that goes beyond the superficiality of physical aesthetics. Ultimately, holistic fitness is a lifestyle that invites individuals to thrive in every dimension of their existence.

The holistic perspective on physical activity

Engaging in physical activity is not just a routine task; it is a holistic commitment to the well-being of both body and mind. The holistic perspective on physical activity transcends the conventional idea of exercise as a mere means to maintain physical fitness. It encompasses a comprehensive approach that acknowledges the interconnectedness of physical, mental, and emotional health.

From a physical standpoint, regular activity is the cornerstone of maintaining a healthy body. It strengthens muscles, improves cardiovascular function, and enhances flexibility. Beyond the aesthetic benefits, physical health is intricately linked to our overall vitality. It boosts the immune system, regulates weight, and promotes longevity.

Embracing a holistic view recognizes that physical activity is not just a measure of aesthetics but a profound investment in our long-term health.

Yet, the holistic perspective goes beyond the physical realm. Physical activity is an invaluable tool for nurturing mental well-being. It is a potent stress-reliever, releasing endorphins that act as natural mood elevators. Regular exercise has been linked to improved cognitive function, enhanced focus, and a reduced risk of mental health disorders. The holistic approach acknowledges the symbiotic relationship between the body and mind, understanding that a healthy body is fundamental to a sound mental state.

Moreover, the holistic perspective on physical activity encompasses emotional and spiritual dimensions. Engaging in activities that bring joy, whether it's dancing, hiking, or practicing yoga, contributes to emotional balance. Physical activity becomes a form of self-expression and a medium for connecting with one's inner self. It fosters a sense of purpose and fulfillment, creating a positive feedback loop that extends beyond the gym or exercise routine.

In the holistic view, physical activity is not confined to a specific duration or type. It becomes a seamless integration into daily life – a walk in the park, a leisurely bike ride, or even mindful stretching. The emphasis is on consistency and sustainability rather than rigid adherence to a specific regimen. This aligns with the understanding that physical well-being is an ongoing journey rather than a destination.

In summary, the holistic perspective on physical activity is a paradigm shift from a narrow focus on exercise routines to a broader commitment to overall well-being. It recognizes the interconnectedness of physical, mental, emotional, and even spiritual dimensions. Embracing this holistic approach to physical activity is an investment in a healthier, happier, and more fulfilling life. It's a recognition that taking care of our bodies is not a chore but a celebration of the incredible vessel that carries us through life.

Embracing a holistic perspective on physical activity goes beyond the mere pursuit of fitness; it encapsulates a comprehensive approach to well-being that extends to the physical, mental, and emotional realms of our lives. In this paradigm, physical activity is not just a means to an end but an integral component of a harmonious and fulfilling lifestyle.

Physical Aspect:

At its core, physical activity contributes to the maintenance and enhancement of bodily functions. Regular exercise strengthens muscles, improves cardiovascular health, and promotes flexibility. It is the cornerstone of weight management, aiding in the prevention of chronic conditions such as obesity, diabetes, and cardiovascular diseases. From vigorous workouts to mindful movements like yoga, the physical aspect of holistic physical activity encompasses a diverse spectrum of exercises tailored to individual needs and preferences.

Mental Well-being:

The benefits extend beyond the physical domain, influencing mental well-being profoundly. Engaging in physical activity triggers the release of endorphins, the feel-good hormones, which contribute to reduced stress and anxiety. It acts as a natural mood booster and is often recommended as an adjunct therapy for managing conditions like depression. Additionally, the cognitive benefits of regular physical activity are increasingly recognized, with research indicating improvements in memory, attention, and overall cognitive function.

Emotional Balance:

Holistic physical activity fosters emotional equilibrium by providing a constructive outlet for stress and pent-up emotions. The rhythmic nature of certain exercises, coupled with the meditative aspects of mindful practices, contributes to emotional grounding. Regular physical activity has been linked to enhanced self-esteem and a more positive self-image, creating a solid foundation for emotional well-being.

Social Connectivity:

Physical activity often extends beyond solitary pursuits, becoming a vehicle for social interaction and connectivity. Group fitness classes, team sports, or even communal walks offer opportunities for social engagement, fostering a sense of community and support. This social dimension contributes to holistic well-being, addressing the human need for connection and belonging.

Lifestyle Integration:

A holistic perspective on physical activity involves integrating movement seamlessly into daily life. This extends beyond scheduled workouts to encompass active commuting, taking the stairs, or incorporating movement breaks into a sedentary work routine. This approach recognizes that physical activity is not confined to the gym but is a dynamic and fluid aspect of our daily existence.

In essence, the holistic perspective on physical activity recognizes that our bodies are not isolated entities but integral components of a complex system that includes mind, emotions, and social connections. By approaching physical activity holistically, we unlock its full potential as a catalyst for a vibrant, balanced, and fulfilling life. It becomes a journey of self-discovery, self-care, and holistic well-being, transcending the boundaries of conventional fitness paradigms.

Integrating exercise routines for body, mind, and spirit.

In the pursuit of holistic well-being, the integration of exercise routines for the body, mind, and spirit stands as a powerful cornerstone. This approach recognizes the interconnected nature of our physical, mental, and spiritual aspects, acknowledging that true health and vitality are not achieved in isolation but through a harmonious balance. Let's delve into the multifaceted benefits and considerations associated with this comprehensive approach to fitness.

Body:

Physical exercise is often the first aspect that comes to mind when considering health, and rightfully so. Engaging in regular exercise

routines enhance cardiovascular health, strengthens muscles, improves flexibility, and contributes to weight management. It is the cornerstone of a healthy body, fostering resilience, and preventing various ailments. Whether it's cardiovascular workouts, strength training, or flexibility exercises, the body thrives when it is consistently and holistically engaged.

Moreover, the body is not a separate entity from the mind and spirit. Physical activity has been proven to release endorphins, neurotransmitters that act as natural mood lifters. This connection between physical exercise and mental well-being is a testament to the profound impact a holistic approach can have on overall health.

Mind:

Exercise is not solely a physical endeavor; it is a powerful tool for nurturing mental wellness. Regular physical activity has been linked to improved cognitive function, enhanced memory, and increased creativity. The rhythmic and repetitive nature of certain exercises, such as running or swimming, can induce a meditative state, promoting mental clarity and stress relief.

Incorporating mind-focused exercises, such as yoga or tai chi, further amplifies the mental benefits. These practices not only improve physical flexibility and balance but also cultivate mindfulness, encouraging individuals to be present in the moment and connect with their inner selves.

Spirit:

The spiritual dimension of exercise extends beyond the conventional understanding of the term. It involves fostering a sense of purpose, connection, and alignment with one's core values. Engaging in activities that bring joy, whether it's dancing, hiking, or any form of movement that resonates with the individual, can be a deeply spiritual experience.

Mindful exercises that involve intentional breathing and focus, like meditation or qigong, provide a bridge to the spiritual realm. They create an avenue for self-reflection, inner peace, and a heightened sense of awareness. The integration of spiritual elements into exercise routines contributes to a profound sense of fulfillment and purpose.

Integrating exercise routines for the body, mind, and spirit is a holistic approach to well-being that recognizes the interconnected nature of our being. By nurturing these dimensions concurrently, individuals can experience not only physical vitality but also mental clarity, emotional resilience, and a deeper connection to their inner selves. It's a journey of self-discovery and self-care that goes beyond the confines of a gym, reaching into the realms of mental and spiritual flourishing.

Highlighting the benefits of holistic fitness for overall wellness:

In the pursuit of a fulfilling and healthy life, the concept of holistic fitness emerges as a guiding philosophy that transcends conventional approaches. Holistic fitness is a comprehensive and integrated approach to wellness that goes beyond mere physical exercise, acknowledging the intricate connection between the mind, body, and spirit. It champions a lifestyle that fosters balance, sustainability, and overall well-being.

At the core of holistic fitness lies the understanding that the body is a complex system, intricately connected to mental and emotional states. Traditional fitness often focuses solely on physical exercise, neglecting the profound impact of mental and emotional health on one's overall wellness. Holistic fitness, however, recognizes that achieving true well-being requires nurturing every aspect of our being.

One of the paramount benefits of holistic fitness is its ability to foster a harmonious relationship between the mind and body. Regular exercise, mindful practices, and stress-reducing activities work synergistically to promote mental clarity, emotional resilience, and a heightened sense of self-awareness. This integration is crucial for not only managing stress but also for preventing the development of chronic conditions associated with modern-day living.

Furthermore, holistic fitness emphasizes the importance of nourishing the body with wholesome nutrition. It transcends the restrictive nature of fad diets and instead advocates for a balanced and sustainable approach to eating. By recognizing the significance of quality nutrients, hydration, and mindful eating practices, holistic fitness becomes a catalyst for optimal physical health and vitality.

Beyond the physical and mental realms, holistic fitness extends its reach to spiritual well-being. It invites individuals to explore practices that connect them with a sense of purpose, inner peace, and a deeper understanding of their place in the world. Whether through meditation, yoga, or other spiritual practices, holistic fitness becomes a transformative journey that enriches the soul and contributes to a more meaningful and fulfilling life.

The holistic approach to fitness also acknowledges the interconnectedness of the individual with their environment. Engaging in outdoor activities, cultivating a connection with nature, and adopting sustainable practices become integral components of holistic fitness. This not only enhances physical fitness but also fosters an appreciation for the interconnectedness of all living things.

In essence, holistic fitness is a multifaceted approach to wellness that promotes balance, resilience, and longevity. It recognizes that true health is not achieved through isolated efforts but through a holistic integration of physical, mental, emotional, and spiritual well-being. By embracing the principles of holistic fitness, individuals can experience a profound transformation that extends far beyond the confines of traditional fitness routines, ultimately leading to a life of vibrancy, purpose, and holistic wellness.

In the quest for optimal well-being, holistic fitness emerges as a comprehensive and transformative approach that extends far beyond mere physical exercise. It's a philosophy that encompasses the entirety of an individual's health—mind, body, and spirit. This holistic perspective recognizes the interconnectedness of various aspects of wellness and emphasizes the symbiotic relationship between physical health, mental clarity, and emotional balance.

Physical Well-being:

At the core of holistic fitness lies a commitment to physical health that goes beyond the superficial. It's not just about sculpting the body but fostering vitality and resilience. Regular exercise, incorporating a mix of cardiovascular activities, strength training, and flexibility exercises, is the cornerstone. This multifaceted approach promotes cardiovascular health, enhances muscular strength and flexibility, and contributes to weight management.

Mental Clarity and Cognitive Function:

Holistic fitness recognizes the profound impact of physical activity on mental health. Engaging in regular exercise releases endorphins, the body's natural mood enhancers, contributing to reduced stress levels and enhanced mental clarity. The improved circulation of oxygen to the brain supports cognitive function, positively influencing memory, focus, and overall mental acuity.

Emotional Balance:

In the pursuit of holistic fitness, emotional well-being takes center stage. Regular physical activity is linked to the release of neurotransmitters like serotonin, which plays a crucial role in mood regulation. Holistic fitness practices often incorporate mind-body exercises such as yoga and meditation, promoting mindfulness and emotional balance. These practices empower individuals to navigate life's challenges with greater resilience and emotional intelligence.

Nutritional Harmony:

Holistic fitness extends its reach to nutrition, recognizing that a well-balanced diet is integral to overall health. It's not about restrictive diets but about nourishing the body with wholesome, nutrient-dense foods. The emphasis is on mindful eating, fostering a positive relationship with food that supports sustained energy levels and promotes internal harmony.

Stress Reduction and Sleep Quality:

One of the notable benefits of holistic fitness

is its impact on stress reduction. Physical activity helps the body metabolize stress hormones, promoting a sense of calm. Combined with mindfulness practices, it contributes to improved sleep quality. Quality sleep is a cornerstone of holistic wellness, facilitating recovery, and ensuring the body's ability to regenerate and heal.

Social and Environmental Wellness:

Beyond individual well-being, holistic fitness acknowledges the importance of social connections and environmental awareness. Group fitness activities and community engagement foster a sense of belonging and support, contributing to mental and emotional wellness. Additionally, outdoor activities promote a connection with nature, emphasizing the significance of a balanced and sustainable relationship with the environment.

In essence, holistic fitness is a transformative journey that recognizes the multidimensional nature of well-being. It's not a one-size-fits-all approach but a personalized and sustainable lifestyle that considers the unique needs of each individual. By embracing the interconnectedness of physical, mental, emotional, and social aspects of health, holistic fitness becomes a powerful catalyst for achieving lasting wellness and vitality.

The Healing Power of Nature

In the cacophony of modern life, the healing power of nature emerges as a silent yet profound force, weaving its therapeutic magic on the tapestry of our well-being. Nature, with its serene landscapes, lush greenery, and the harmonious melody of birdsong, beckons us to pause, breathe, and immerse ourselves in its calming embrace.

From time immemorial, humanity has sought solace in the natural world. There's an inherent connection between us and the elements – a connection that extends beyond the superficiality of day-to-day stressors. In the quiet rustle of leaves or the rhythmic lapping of waves against the shore, there exists a healing energy that transcends the tangible.

The healing power of nature isn't just a concept; it's a visceral experience. Scientific studies corroborate what our instincts have long intuited: spending time in nature is associated with reduced stress levels, improved mood, and enhanced overall well-being. The mere act of being surrounded by trees, breathing in fresh air, and absorbing the warmth of natural sunlight can have transformative effects on our mental and physical health.

Nature provides a sanctuary for the mind, a refuge from the relentless demands of the digital age. In its expansive quietude, we find an opportunity to recalibrate, to attune ourselves to the gentle rhythms of the earth. A walk in the woods becomes more than just a stroll; it becomes a pilgrimage to rediscover our innate connection with the natural world.

Moreover, the healing power of nature isn't confined to the exterior landscape alone. It extends to the depths of our internal landscapes, offering a balm for the soul.

Nature serves as a catalyst for introspection, encouraging us to delve into the recesses of our thoughts and emotions. It becomes a mirror, reflecting the ebb and flow of our innermost feelings.

In an era dominated by concrete jungles and technology-driven lives, the imperative to reconnect with nature becomes increasingly crucial. The healing power of nature is a call to return to our roots, to rediscover the simplicity and authenticity that nature effortlessly exudes. It's an invitation to be present, to engage our senses, and to witness the profound beauty that unfolds when we pause and listen to the whispers of the natural world.

So, whether it's the hushed serenity of a forest, the rhythmic cadence of ocean waves, or the vibrant hues of a sunset, let us embrace the healing power of nature. In its embrace, we find restoration, rejuvenation, and a timeless reminder of the delicate dance between humanity and the Earth – a dance that, when honored, can profoundly enrich the tapestry of our lives.

Connecting with nature for holistic well-being

Immersing oneself in nature is like hitting the reset button for the soul. It's an opportunity to step away from the demands of daily life, disconnect from the constant buzz of screens, and reconnect with the natural rhythm of the earth. The benefits extend far beyond mere relaxation; they encompass a profound sense of holistic well-being.

One of the key facets of connecting with nature is the restoration it provides for our mental health. The calmness of a forest, the rhythmic sound of ocean waves, or the gentle rustling of leaves in a park – these natural environments have an incredible capacity to alleviate stress, anxiety, and mental fatigue. It's a chance to unplug from the digital noise and tune into the soothing melodies of the natural world.

Moreover, nature offers a sanctuary for introspection and mindfulness. In the midst of towering trees or expansive landscapes, individuals often find clarity of thought and a space for reflection. It's a setting conducive to contemplation, self-discovery, and the cultivation of a mindful presence in the current moment.

The physical benefits of connecting with nature are equally compelling. Outdoor activities like hiking, walking, or even a simple picnic encourage movement, promoting physical health and vitality. Breathing in fresh, unpolluted air and absorbing natural sunlight contribute to improved immune function and enhanced overall well-being.

Beyond the individual, nature has the power to foster a sense of community and interconnectedness. Shared outdoor experiences create bonds, whether it's a family hike, a community gardening project, or a group outing to a natural landmark. These shared connections enhance social well-being, contributing to a sense of belonging and support.

As we immerse ourselves in the natural world, we also gain a profound appreciation for the environment. This heightened awareness often leads to a more conscious and sustainable lifestyle, fostering a sense of responsibility towards the planet we call home.

In essence, connecting with nature is not merely a leisurely activity; it's a holistic journey towards well-being that encompasses the physical, mental, and social dimensions of our lives. It's a reminder that, in the midst of our bustling lives, the antidote to stress and the pathway to holistic well-being may be just a step outside our door, surrounded by the timeless wonders of the natural world, reconnecting with nature stands as a powerful antidote for achieving holistic well-being. The natural world has a profound impact on our physical, mental, and emotional health, offering a sanctuary where we can find balance and renewal.

Nature's Therapeutic Influence:

Engaging with nature is not just a leisure activity; it's a therapeutic journey. The sensory experiences – the rustling of leaves, the scent of pine, the warmth of sunlight – resonate with our senses, triggering a cascade of positive physiological responses. Scientific studies affirm that exposure to nature reduces stress, lowers blood pressure, and enhances overall mood. It's a natural prescription for healing the mind and body.

Emotional Resonance:

Nature has an unparalleled ability to evoke emotions and connect us to something greater than ourselves. Whether it's the awe-inspiring grandeur of a mountain range, the serenity of a babbling brook, or the vibrant hues of a sunset, these experiences tap into our emotional reservoir, fostering a profound sense of peace, gratitude, and joy.

Mindful Presence in Nature:

Connecting with nature isn't just about being

physically present; it's about cultivating mindfulness. When we immerse ourselves in nature, we're encouraged to engage our senses fully. Observing the intricate details of a flower, listening to the melody of birdsong, or feeling the earth beneath our feet – these moments anchor us in the present, providing a respite from the pressures of daily life.

Physical Well-Being:

Nature beckons us to move, breathe, and embrace a more active lifestyle. Whether it's a hike through a lush forest or a gentle stroll in a city park, the act of being outdoors promotes physical activity, supporting cardiovascular health, reducing sedentary behavior, and enhancing overall well-being.

Connection to the Seasons:

Nature's cyclical rhythms mirror the ebb and flow of our lives. Observing the changing seasons – the blossoming of spring, the warmth of summer, the transition of autumn, and the quiet reflection of winter – provides a sense of continuity and connection to the natural cycles that govern our existence.

Cultivating a Sense of Wonder:

Nature sparks curiosity and wonder, inviting us to explore and marvel at the mysteries of the world. This sense of awe fosters a childlike curiosity that can be transformative, encouraging us to question, learn, and remain open to the magic that surrounds us.

Building Community and Social Bonds:

Nature acts as a unifying force, bringing people together. Whether through outdoor activities, community gardening, or simply sharing a picnic in a park, nature provides a backdrop for forging meaningful connections. These shared experiences contribute to a sense of belonging and social cohesion.

In essence, connecting with nature isn't just a leisurely pursuit; it's a holistic journey that encompasses the physical, emotional, and spiritual dimensions of our well-being. It's a conscious choice to step outside, breathe in the fresh air, and embrace the beauty that surrounds us – a choice that holds the key to a more balanced, centered, and fulfilled life.

Exploring ecotherapy, outdoor activities, and the impact of nature on health

The therapeutic power of nature stands as a sanctuary waiting to be explored. Ecotherapy, an evolving field that combines psychological principles with outdoor activities, has emerged as a profound means of improving mental and emotional well-being. The profound impact of nature on our health is a topic that transcends mere scientific analysis; it touches the essence of what it means to be human. Studies have consistently shown that spending time outdoors, engaging in activities immersed in the natural world, can significantly alleviate stress, reduce anxiety, and even contribute to better overall mental health.

Ecotherapy embraces a holistic approach, recognizing the interconnectedness between human well-being and the environment. Whether it's a serene walk in the woods, gardening, or simply basking in the beauty of a natural landscape, these activities serve as potent antidotes to the stresses of daily life. Nature becomes a therapeutic canvas, a backdrop against which individuals can recalibrate their mental and emotional states.

The healing power of nature is not a new concept; it's deeply ingrained in our history and cultural traditions. Indigenous practices, ancient philosophies, and even literary works have celebrated the symbiotic relationship between humanity and the natural world. Ecotherapy taps into this innate connection, urging individuals to step outside, breathe in the fresh air, and rediscover the simplicity and beauty that nature effortlessly provides.

Note also that the impact of nature on health extends beyond psychological benefits. Physical activities conducted in natural settings contribute to improved cardiovascular health, increased vitamin D intake, and a bolstered immune system. The harmonious synergy between the mind and body is evident when one engages in outdoor pursuits, whether it's hiking, cycling, or simply enjoying the serenity of a natural setting.

As we delve deeper into the exploration of ecotherapy and outdoor activities, it's crucial to acknowledge the growing body of evidence supporting the positive impact of nature on specific mental health conditions. Nature-based interventions have shown promise in alleviating symptoms of depression, anxiety, and attention deficit disorders. The immersive experience of being surrounded by natural elements fosters a sense of calmness and connection that can be transformative for those grappling with mental health challenges.

Moreover, ecotherapy isn't confined to remote wilderness areas. Urban green spaces, community gardens, and even potted plants on a balcony can serve as conduits for reaping the benefits of nature on health. The inclusivity of ecotherapy emphasizes that the healing power of nature is accessible to all, irrespective of one's geographical location or lifestyle.

In conclusion, exploring ecotherapy and embracing outdoor activities isn't just about stepping outside; it's a profound journey of rediscovery. It's about reconnecting with the fundamental elements that sustain us and recognizing that, in the grand tapestry of life, nature plays a central role in promoting holistic well-being. So, let us step into the open embrace of the outdoors, let nature be our guide, and let the impact on our health be a testament to the enduring alliance between humanity and the natural world.

CHAPTER SIX:

Holistic Approaches to Mental Health:

In our fast-paced world, where stress and anxiety often seem like unwelcome companions, exploring holistic approaches to mental health has become increasingly vital. Holistic mental health care recognizes the intricate connection between the mind, body, and spirit, aiming to foster balance and well-being on all fronts.

Understanding Holistic Mental Health:

The Mind-Body Connection:

Holistic approaches emphasize the profound interplay between mental and physical health. It acknowledges that mental well-being is not isolated but intricately linked to our physical state. Practices like mindfulness, meditation, and yoga are woven into the fabric of holistic mental health care, fostering harmony between the mind and body.

Nutritional Support:

A crucial element often overlooked is the impact of nutrition on mental health. Holistic approaches advocate for a well-balanced and nutrient-rich diet, recognizing the influence of food on mood and cognitive function. The gut-brain connection is explored, emphasizing the role of a healthy digestive system in maintaining mental equilibrium.

Mindfulness and Meditation:

Central to holistic mental health is the cultivation of mindfulness – the practice of being present in the moment without judgment. Meditation, whether guided or self-directed, becomes a powerful tool to quiet the mind, reduce stress, and enhance emotional resilience. These practices not only provide relief from the demands of modern life but also contribute to long-term mental clarity.

Physical Activity and Mental Wellness:

Exercise, beyond its physical benefits, emerges as a cornerstone of holistic mental health. Whether through aerobic activities, strength training, or simply connecting with nature through a walk, physical activity releases endorphins and fosters a positive mood. The holistic perspective acknowledges that a healthy body contributes significantly to a healthy mind.

Holistic Therapies:

Art and Music Therapy:

Expressive therapies like art and music offer avenues for self-expression and emotional release. Holistic mental health recognizes the therapeutic power of creative outlets, tapping into the healing potential of artistic endeavors to promote mental and emotional well-being.

Acupuncture and Traditional Healing Practices:

Holistic approaches often integrate traditional healing practices, such as acupuncture, herbal medicine, or Ayurveda. These methods consider the individual as a whole and address imbalances not just at the symptom level but at the root, promoting a comprehensive approach to mental health.

Energy Healing and Spirituality:

For many, holistic mental health extends beyond the physical and delves into the realm of spirituality. Practices like energy healing, Reiki, or mindfulness-based spiritual practices become integral components, allowing individuals to explore the connection between their mental well-being and their sense of purpose and spirituality.

Embracing a Holistic Lifestyle:

Holistic Sleep Hygiene:

Quality sleep is a fundamental pillar of mental health. Holistic approaches emphasize the importance of sleep hygiene, incorporating practices that promote restorative sleep, such as creating a calming bedtime routine and optimizing the sleep environment.

Cultivating Healthy Relationships:

The holistic perspective acknowledges the impact of social connections on mental health. Nurturing healthy relationships, setting boundaries, and fostering positive social interactions become essential components of mental well-being.

Stress Management and Holistic Therapies:

Stress is an inevitable part of life, but holistic approaches equip individuals with a toolbox of techniques for managing stress. From progressive muscle relaxation to aromatherapy, these therapies address stressors on multiple levels, promoting overall mental resilience.

In the tapestry of holistic mental health, each thread represents a unique aspect of an individual's well-being. By recognizing the interconnectedness of the mind, body, and spirit, holistic approaches empower individuals to take an active role in their mental health journey. It's an invitation to explore a diverse array of practices, therapies, and lifestyle choices, forging a path toward lasting balance and mental flourishing. As we embrace holistic mental health, we embark on a journey not only to alleviate symptoms but to cultivate a richer, more fulfilling life.

Exploring alternative therapies, counseling, and mindfulness for mental well-being

Exploring alternative therapies, counseling, and mindfulness offers a holistic framework for individuals seeking not just relief but a deeper understanding of their mental health.

Alternative Therapies:

Beyond conventional treatments, alternative therapies provide a diverse spectrum of options for mental well-being. Practices such as acupuncture, aromatherapy, and herbal supplements are gaining popularity for their potential in alleviating symptoms of anxiety and depression. These modalities often focus on restoring balance and harmony within the body, recognizing the intricate connection between mental and physical health.

Counseling Services:

Counseling emerges as a cornerstone in the journey toward mental wellness. Various therapeutic approaches, such as cognitive-behavioral therapy (CBT), dialectical behavior therapy (DBT), and psychoanalysis, offer tailored strategies for addressing a range of mental health concerns. Professional counselors provide a safe space for individuals to explore and navigate their thoughts and emotions, fostering self-awareness and facilitating positive behavioral changes.

Mindfulness Practices:

At the heart of mental well-being lies the practice of mindfulness. Drawing inspiration from ancient contemplative traditions, mindfulness involves cultivating awareness of the present moment without judgment. Mindfulness meditation, yoga, and mindful breathing are powerful tools that promote emotional regulation, stress reduction, and enhanced overall mental resilience. These practices empower individuals to develop a more compassionate and accepting relationship with their thoughts and emotions.

Holistic Approaches:

The integration of alternative therapies, counseling, and mindfulness forms a holistic approach that acknowledges the interconnectedness of mind, body, and spirit. Holistic mental health embraces lifestyle factors such as nutrition, exercise, and sleep, recognizing their profound impact on emotional well-being. This comprehensive approach aims not just to treat symptoms but to address the root causes of mental health challenges.

Personalized Well-Being Plans:

One of the strengths of exploring alternative therapies, counseling, and mindfulness is the ability to create personalized well-being plans. Recognizing that individuals respond differently to various interventions, this approach allows for customization based on preferences, cultural backgrounds, and individual needs. Personalized plans ensure that individuals actively engage in their mental health journey, fostering a sense of empowerment and ownership.

Summarily, the exploration of alternative therapies, counseling, and mindfulness reflects a paradigm shift in how we approach mental well-being. By embracing a spectrum of modalities that address the diverse facets of human experience, individuals can embark on a transformative journey toward understanding, resilience, and sustained mental health. This holistic approach recognizes that mental well-being is not a destination but a continuous, dynamic process of self-discovery and growth.

CHAPTER SEVEN:

Spiritual Wellness and Connection

Beyond the tangible aspects of existence, the realm of spirituality invites us to explore the depths of our inner selves and establish a connection with something greater than our individuality.

Understanding Spiritual Wellness:

Spiritual wellness is a multifaceted concept that transcends religious affiliations. It encompasses a deep sense of purpose, meaning, and connection to the universe. At its core, spiritual wellness involves aligning one's values with actions, finding inner peace, and nurturing a harmonious relationship with the world.

Connecting with the Self:

Central to spiritual wellness is the journey inward – a process of self-discovery and introspection. This involves understanding one's beliefs, values, and the principles that guide one's life. Through practices like meditation, mindfulness, and reflection, individuals can forge a stronger connection with their inner selves, fostering a sense of clarity and purpose.

Harmony with the Universe:

Spiritual wellness extends beyond the self to encompass a connection with the universe or a higher power. This connection is not confined to a specific religious doctrine but rather encourages individuals to recognize their place in the grand tapestry of existence. Whether through nature, art, or contemplative practices, the goal is to experience a sense of awe and reverence for the interconnectedness of all things.

Mind-Body-Spirit Integration:

A holistic approach to spiritual wellness involves recognizing the intricate interplay between the mind, body, and spirit. Practices like yoga, tai chi, or other mindful physical activities can facilitate this integration, promoting a sense of balance and overall well-being.

Cultivating Gratitude and Compassion:

Gratitude is a cornerstone of spiritual wellness. Acknowledging and appreciating the blessings in one's life fosters a positive mindset and a deeper connection to the present moment. Similarly, compassion, both for oneself and others, is a powerful tool for nurturing spiritual well-being. Acts of kindness and empathy contribute to a sense of interconnectedness with humanity.

Finding Meaning in Adversity:

Spiritual wellness provides a framework for finding meaning in the face of adversity. It offers solace and resilience during challenging times by encouraging individuals to view difficulties as opportunities for growth and transformation.

Embracing Spiritual Practices:

There is a myriad of spiritual practices that individuals can explore to enhance their spiritual wellness. These may include prayer, meditation, journaling, attending spiritual gatherings, or engaging in rituals that resonate with personal beliefs.

In essence, the pursuit of spiritual wellness and connection is a deeply personal and ongoing journey. It involves an exploration of the self, an acknowledgment of the interconnected nature of existence, and a commitment to nurturing a sense of purpose and meaning. As individuals delve into this transformative process, they may discover that spiritual wellness not only enhances their personal well-being but also contributes to a more compassionate and harmonious world.

The significance of spirituality in holistic health

Holistic health, a concept that encompasses the well-being of the mind, body, and spirit, has gained increasing recognition in contemporary wellness discussions. Among the multifaceted elements contributing to holistic health, spirituality holds a profound and indispensable place. The integration of spirituality into one's life can significantly impact overall well-being, fostering a sense of connection, purpose, and resilience.

Spirituality, in the context of holistic health, extends beyond traditional religious practices. It encompasses a deep sense of inner peace, purpose, and interconnectedness with oneself, others, and the universe. Here's a comprehensive exploration of the significance of spirituality in holistic health:

1. Inner Peace and Emotional Well-being:

Spirituality provides sanctuary for cultivating

inner peace. Practices such as meditation, mindfulness, and prayer offer individuals a space to connect with their inner selves, promoting emotional balance. This sense of tranquility becomes a cornerstone for managing stress, anxiety, and other emotional challenges, contributing significantly to mental and emotional well-being.

2. Purpose and Meaning:

A spiritual foundation adds depth and meaning to life. It helps individuals discover or reaffirm their sense of purpose, guiding them toward activities and goals aligned with their core values. This sense of purpose becomes a driving force for making healthier lifestyle choices, fostering a holistic approach to well-being.

3. Resilience in the Face of Challenges:

Spirituality provides a reservoir of strength during challenging times. Belief systems and spiritual practices offer a framework for coping with adversity, loss, and uncertainty. The resilience cultivated through spirituality becomes a vital asset in navigating life's ups and downs, contributing to a more robust holistic health profile.

4. Connection and Community:

Spirituality often involves a sense of connection – not only with oneself but also with others and the wider world. Engaging in spiritual communities or practices encourages a supportive network, reducing feelings of isolation. This sense of belonging contributes to emotional health, reinforcing the idea that individuals are not alone on their journey to holistic well-being.

5. Mind-Body Harmony:

Spirituality is intimately connected with the mind-body relationship. Practices like yoga and tai chi, deeply rooted in spiritual traditions, emphasize the connection between mental and physical health. The harmony achieved through these practices supports overall wellness, promoting flexibility, strength, and mental clarity.

6. Enhanced Quality of Relationships:

Spirituality fosters qualities such as compassion, empathy, and forgiveness. These attributes contribute to healthier and more fulfilling relationships, creating a positive ripple effect on overall well-being. Nurturing spiritual connections often translates into improved communication, understanding, and support within interpersonal relationships.

7. Encouraging Healthy Habits:

Many spiritual traditions promote a mindful and intentional approach to daily living. This mindfulness extends to choices around nutrition, exercise, and self-care. Integrating spirituality into one's life often leads to a heightened awareness of the body's needs, encouraging individuals to adopt healthier lifestyle habits that contribute to holistic health.

In a nutshell spirituality serves as a cornerstone in the holistic health framework, providing a profound and multifaceted impact on the mind, body, and spirit. As individuals explore and nurture their spiritual well-being, they discover a path to a more balanced, purposeful, and resilient life. The significance of spirituality in holistic health lies in its ability to enrich every facet of the human experience, promoting a harmonious and fulfilling existence.

Exploring spiritual practices, meditation, and their impact on overall wellness.

In the quest for holistic well-being, the exploration of spiritual practices and meditation emerges as a profound journey into the depths of the self. These practices, deeply rooted in ancient traditions and philosophies, go beyond the physical realm, seeking to nourish the mind, body, and soul in a harmonious union.

Spiritual Practices:

At the core of spiritual practices lies a diverse tapestry of rituals, traditions, and disciplines. Whether rooted in religious traditions, mindfulness techniques, or personal philosophies, these practices share a common thread—connecting individuals with a sense of purpose, inner peace, and transcendence.

From prayer and chanting to contemplative walks in nature, these rituals serve as conduits for fostering a deeper understanding of the self and the universe.

Meditation:

Meditation, a timeless practice with roots in various cultures, emerges as a transformative tool in the pursuit of inner balance. It extends an invitation to quiet the incessant chatter of the mind, providing a sanctuary where one can delve into the present moment. From mindfulness meditation to guided visualizations, the diverse array of techniques empowers individuals to cultivate a heightened state of awareness, reduce stress, and foster emotional resilience.

Impact on Overall Wellness:

The profound impact of spiritual practices and meditation on overall wellness is multifaceted, influencing the physical, mental, and spiritual dimensions of our existence.

- **Mental Clarity and Focus:**
  - Through the stillness cultivated in meditation, individuals often find enhanced mental clarity and improved focus. This heightened awareness enables better decision-making, problem-solving, and an overall sharpening of cognitive functions.
- **Emotional Well-Being:**
  - Spiritual practices often involve exploring the depths of one's

emotions, fostering self-awareness and emotional intelligence. Meditation, in particular, provides a sanctuary for processing and understanding emotions, leading to greater emotional resilience and balance.

- **Stress Reduction:**
  - The mindfulness inherent in spiritual practices and meditation acts as a powerful antidote to stress. By anchoring attention to the present moment, these practices alleviate the burden of past regrets and future anxieties, promoting a profound sense of peace.
- **Physical Health:**
  - Scientific studies increasingly highlight the positive impact of

meditation on physical health. From reduced blood pressure to enhanced immune system function, the mind–body connection cultivated through these practices contributes to a comprehensive approach to well–being.

- **Enhanced Spirituality:**
  - For many, the exploration of spiritual practices is a journey towards a deeper connection with their spiritual selves or a higher power. This connection often brings about a sense of purpose, inner fulfillment, and a profound understanding of the interconnectedness of all life.

In conclusion, the exploration of spiritual practices and meditation transcends the boundaries of conventional wellness approaches. It invites individuals to embark on an introspective journey, cultivating a state of balance, peace, and interconnectedness that extends far beyond the physical realm. As we delve into these practices, we find not just moments of tranquility but keys to unlocking the vast potential of our overall well-being.

Nurturing spiritual well-being for a balanced and fulfilling life

Beyond the tangible aspects of our daily routines and material pursuits, there exists a profound need to connect with the spiritual dimensions of our being – a realm that transcends the immediate and touches the very core of who we are.

Understanding Spiritual Well-being:

Spiritual well-being encompasses more than religious affiliations; it's a deeply personal journey that involves connecting with a sense of purpose, inner peace, and transcendence. It involves aligning our values, beliefs, and actions with a higher sense of meaning. This spiritual aspect of life is the compass that guides us when faced with challenges, provides solace during turbulent times, and infuses our lives with a profound sense of fulfillment.

Connection to Inner Self:

Nurturing spiritual well-being involves delving into the depths of our inner selves. It's about self-reflection, mindfulness, and creating a space for contemplation. Through practices like meditation, prayer, or simply moments of stillness, we tap into a reservoir of inner wisdom, gaining clarity and a heightened awareness of our true selves.

Cultivating Gratitude and Positivity:

Spiritual well-being thrives in an environment of gratitude and positivity. Acknowledging the blessings in our lives, no matter how small, fosters a mindset of abundance. This positivity becomes a powerful force, shaping our perceptions, interactions, and responses to the challenges we encounter.

Harmony with Nature and the Universe:

Connecting with our spiritual side often involves recognizing our place within the larger tapestry of existence. Whether through communing with nature, stargazing, or contemplating the vastness of the universe, we find a sense of humility and interconnectedness that transcends the boundaries of our individual lives.

Seeking Meaning and Purpose:

A life rich in spiritual well-being is one anchored in meaning and purpose. It's about aligning our actions with our values and contributing to something greater than ourselves. This quest for purpose becomes a driving force, infusing our endeavors with passion and significance.

Practices for Spiritual Nourishment:

Nurturing spiritual well-being encompasses a myriad of practices. For some, it may involve regular attendance at religious services, while for others, it could be found in the pages of sacred texts, philosophical readings, or moments of quiet reflection. Engaging in activities that bring joy, practicing compassion, and fostering connections with others all contribute to a spiritually fulfilling life.

Balancing the Material and Spiritual:

In the pursuit of a balanced and fulfilling life, it's crucial to strike a harmonious balance between the material and spiritual aspects. While material pursuits provide a sense of security and comfort, spiritual well-being offers the compass that guides these pursuits with intention, ensuring they align with our deeper values; nurturing spiritual well-being is an ongoing, dynamic process that evolves as we grow and navigate the complexities of life. It's about finding a sense of peace and purpose that transcends the transient nature of our daily experiences. As we embark on this journey, we discover that spiritual well-being not only enhances our personal fulfillment but also ripples outward, positively influencing the lives of those around us. It becomes the foundation for a truly balanced and deeply fulfilling existence.

CHAPTER EIGHT:

Building Healthy Relationships

Building healthy relationships is a multifaceted and dynamic process that involves a myriad of factors, ranging from effective communication to empathy, trust, and mutual respect. At its core, a healthy relationship is a partnership that nurtures personal growth, happiness, and emotional well-being for all involved.

Communication is Key:

One of the foundational pillars of a healthy relationship is effective communication. This goes beyond mere exchange of words; it involves active listening, understanding, and expressing oneself openly and honestly. Creating a safe space where both parties feel heard and valued fosters a sense of connection and emotional intimacy.

Trust and Transparency:

Trust is the glue that binds relationships together. Building and maintaining trust requires transparency, reliability, and consistency in actions. When individuals feel secure in their relationship, they are more likely to open up, share vulnerabilities, and collaborate in the face of challenges.

Empathy and Understanding:

A healthy relationship thrives on empathy – the ability to understand and share the feelings of another. Cultivating empathy creates an emotional connection, allowing individuals to appreciate each other's perspectives and navigate conflicts with compassion. It fosters an environment where partners feel supported and acknowledged.

Respecting Boundaries:

Respecting each other's boundaries is vital for the health of any relationship. It involves recognizing and honoring personal space, values, and individual aspirations. Establishing clear boundaries promotes autonomy and helps prevent feelings of suffocation or resentment.

Conflict Resolution:

No relationship is without its challenges, but how conflicts are handled can significantly impact its health. Healthy relationships involve constructive conflict resolution, where both parties feel heard and understood. The focus should be on finding solutions rather than placing blame.

Shared Values and Goals:

Aligning values and goals provides a sense of direction and purpose in a relationship. When partners share common values and aspirations, they are more likely to support each other's personal growth and work together towards a shared vision of the future.

Quality Time and Connection:

Investing quality time in a relationship is crucial for building a strong bond. Whether it's through shared activities, meaningful conversations, or simply being present for each other, creating moments of connection reinforces the emotional closeness that sustains a healthy relationship.

Cultivating Positivity:

A positive and nurturing environment is essential for the longevity of a healthy relationship. Expressing appreciation, celebrating successes, and finding joy in shared experiences contribute to an atmosphere that uplifts both partners and strengthens their connection.

In essence, building healthy relationships is an ongoing process that requires commitment, effort, and a genuine desire for mutual well-being. It's about fostering an environment where individuals feel valued, understood, and supported on their respective journeys. As relationships evolve, adapting to the changing needs of each partner and the relationship itself becomes paramount for continued growth and fulfillment.

The role of relationships in holistic health.

In the intricate tapestry of human existence, the role of relationships in holistic health emerges as a central thread, weaving its influence across the realms of physical, mental, and emotional well-being. Beyond the conventional markers of health, the quality of our connections with others becomes a powerful determinant of our overall vitality and flourishing.

At its core, holistic health transcends the narrow confines of physical wellness. It extends its reach to encompass the intricate interplay between mind, body, and spirit. Relationships, whether familial, romantic, or social, serve as conduits through which our innermost selves find expression. The bonds we form and nurture contribute to an ecosystem that either nurtures or hinders our holistic well-being.

Emotional well-being, a cornerstone of holistic health, finds its roots entwined with the fabric of relationships. The warmth of genuine connections provides a sanctuary where emotions can be expressed authentically and received without judgment.

Supportive relationships act as buffers against the storms of life, enhancing resilience and offering solace during challenging times.

In the realm of mental health, the influence of relationships is equally profound. Meaningful connections stimulate cognitive functions, fostering mental agility and creativity. Engaging in deep, meaningful conversations with loved ones can provide intellectual nourishment, challenging our perspectives and broadening our mental horizons. Conversely, toxic relationships can exert a detrimental impact, contributing to stress, anxiety, and even cognitive decline.

Physical health, too, dances in tandem with the quality of our relationships. Research consistently highlights the tangible health benefits of strong social connections. From bolstering immune function to reducing the risk of chronic diseases, the positive impact of robust relationships on physical well-being is undeniable. Shared activities, whether exercise routines or wholesome meals, become avenues through which health is cultivated collectively.

The reciprocity of influence between relationships and holistic health is dynamic. Just as our well-being shapes the quality of our connections, the support and understanding found in relationships reciprocate by enhancing our capacity for holistic flourishing. Shared laughter, empathetic listening, and the sense of belonging that accompanies meaningful relationships contribute to a positive feedback loop, reinforcing the foundation of holistic health.

Conversely, the strains of strained relationships can cast a shadow on our well-being. Unresolved conflicts, toxic dynamics, and a lack of authentic communication can become stressors that seep into the various dimensions of our health. The toll is not merely emotional but extends its tendrils into physical and mental realms, manifesting in ailments and a diminished sense of vitality.

The role of relationships in holistic health is multifaceted and profound. It extends far beyond the confines of emotional bonds to shape our mental, physical, and even spiritual well-being. Nurturing healthy connections becomes not only a source of joy and fulfillment but an indispensable pillar supporting our journey towards holistic health and a flourishing life.

Strategies for cultivating positive connections and managing conflicts

Building and maintaining positive connections with others is a multifaceted process that involves both the art of communication and the ability to navigate conflicts effectively. In various aspects of life, whether personal or professional, the quality of our relationships significantly influences our overall well-being and success. Here, we delve into strategies for cultivating positive connections and managing conflicts to foster meaningful, harmonious interactions.

Cultivating Positive Connections:

Effective Communication: Open and honest

communication serves as the bedrock for positive connections. Actively listen, express your thoughts clearly, and seek to understand others. Foster an environment where individuals feel heard and valued.

Empathy and Understanding: Cultivating empathy allows us to see situations from others' perspectives, fostering a deeper connection. Understand that everyone comes with unique experiences, and acknowledging those differences can strengthen your bonds.

Building Trust: Trust is the cornerstone of any positive relationship. Consistency, reliability, and transparency contribute to the development of trust over time. Be true to your word and demonstrate integrity in your actions.

Shared Values and Interests: Identify common ground and shared interests to create a foundation for positive connections. Engaging in activities or discussions that align with shared values strengthens the bond and creates a sense of belonging.

Encouragement and Support: Positivity thrives in an environment where encouragement and support are present. Celebrate others' successes, provide constructive feedback, and offer a helping hand when needed. A supportive atmosphere fosters positive connections.

Managing Conflicts:

Effective Communication During Conflicts: Conflicts are inevitable, but how we navigate them is key. Foster an environment where individuals feel safe expressing concerns.

Use "I" statements to avoid blame and focus on expressing feelings and needs.

Active Listening: During conflicts, ensure that you actively listen to the other person's perspective. Seek to understand their viewpoint without interrupting. This not only demonstrates respect but also helps in finding common ground.

Seeking Solutions, Not Blame: When conflicts arise, shift the focus from assigning blame to seeking solutions. Collaborate on finding mutually beneficial resolutions rather than dwelling on past grievances.

Emotional Regulation: Conflicts often evoke strong emotions. Learning to regulate your emotions allows for more rational and constructive conversations. Take a moment if needed, and return to the discussion with a calmer demeanor.

Understanding Different Communication Styles: People communicate differently, and conflicts can sometimes arise from misinterpretations. Recognize and appreciate diverse communication styles, adjusting your approach to enhance understanding.

Conflict Resolution Strategies: Familiarize yourself with various conflict resolution strategies, such as compromise, collaboration, or finding common ground. Tailor your approach based on the nature of the conflict and the individuals involved.

The journey towards cultivating positive connections and managing conflicts is a continuous process of self-awareness, effective communication, and a commitment to fostering understanding. By embracing these strategies, you can contribute to building a positive and harmonious environment in both personal and professional spheres of life.

Emphasizing the impact of healthy relationships on overall well-being.

CHAPTER NINE:

Holistic Sleep Hygiene

Achieving a restful and rejuvenating night's sleep extends beyond just the number of hours spent in bed. Holistic sleep hygiene encompasses a comprehensive approach to optimizing the quality and quantity of your sleep, acknowledging that various lifestyle factors influence our ability to rest well. In this exploration of holistic sleep hygiene, we delve into the multifaceted elements that contribute to a truly restorative slumber.

Understanding Sleep Cycles:

Sleep is a dynamic process characterized by distinct cycles, including both rapid eye movement (REM) and non-REM stages. Holistic sleep hygiene recognizes the significance of achieving a balance between these stages to ensure comprehensive restoration for the body and mind.

Creating a Sleep-Inducing Environment:

Consider your sleep environment as a sanctuary for tranquility. This involves addressing factors such as room temperature, lighting, and noise levels. Embrace calming colors, invest in blackout curtains, and explore white noise machines to foster an environment conducive to relaxation.

Establishing Consistent Sleep Patterns:

The body thrives on routine, and sleep is no

exception. Holistic sleep hygiene encourages the establishment of consistent sleep patterns, including regular bedtime and wake-up times. Aligning your sleep schedule with your body's natural circadian rhythm promotes a more harmonious sleep-wake cycle.

Mindful Nutrition for Better Sleep:

Diet plays a crucial role in sleep quality. Holistic sleep hygiene involves mindful nutrition practices, such as avoiding heavy meals close to bedtime and incorporating sleep-promoting foods like almonds, cherries, and fatty fish into your evening routine.

Physical Activity and Sleep:

Regular exercise contributes to overall

well-being, but it also plays a vital role in promoting better sleep. Holistic sleep hygiene encourages a balance of physical activity, emphasizing the importance of consistent exercise without engaging in intense workouts too close to bedtime.

Stress Management Techniques:

Stress can be a significant disruptor of sleep. Holistic sleep hygiene incorporates stress management techniques such as mindfulness, meditation, and deep breathing exercises to cultivate a sense of calm before bedtime.

Digital Detox for Restful Nights:

The pervasive use of electronic devices can interfere with sleep due to the exposure to blue light emitted from screens. Holistic sleep hygiene advises a digital detox before bedtime, limiting screen time and creating a technology-free buffer zone to signal the body that it's time to wind down.

Optimizing Sleep Posture and Comfort:

Investing in a comfortable mattress and pillows that support your preferred sleep position is essential for holistic sleep hygiene. Adequate support for the spine and joints contributes to a more restful and uninterrupted night's sleep.

Hydration for Nighttime Wellness:

Maintaining proper hydration levels throughout the day positively impacts sleep quality. Holistic sleep hygiene involves mindful hydration practices, ensuring you strike a balance to prevent disturbances from midnight trips to the bathroom.

In essence, holistic sleep hygiene is a holistic lifestyle approach that acknowledges the interconnectedness of various factors influencing our sleep. By embracing these principles, individuals can cultivate a sleep environment and routine that not only promotes restful nights but also contributes to overall well-being. Remember, achieving optimal sleep is not a one-size-fits-all endeavor, and adopting a holistic approach allows for personalized adjustments that cater to individual needs and preferences.

Achieving a restful night's sleep is not merely a matter of counting sheep; it involves embracing a comprehensive approach known as Holistic Sleep Hygiene. This concept goes beyond conventional sleep tips and addresses the various interconnected factors that influence the quality of our sleep. By adopting a holistic perspective, individuals can cultivate an environment conducive to rest, foster healthy habits, and ultimately enhance their overall well-being.

Understanding Holistic Sleep Hygiene:

Holistic Sleep Hygiene recognizes that sleep is a multifaceted aspect of our lives, influenced by physical, mental, and environmental factors. It delves into the interconnectedness of these elements, emphasizing a balanced and all-encompassing approach to promote better sleep.

Creating a Sleep-Inducing Environment:

A crucial aspect of Holistic Sleep Hygiene is crafting an environment that signals the body and mind that it's time for rest. This involves considerations such as optimizing bedroom lighting, managing noise levels, and ensuring a comfortable mattress and pillows. By transforming the bedroom into a haven for relaxation, individuals can set the stage for restorative sleep.

Establishing Consistent Sleep Patterns:

Holistic sleep hygiene encourages the establishment of consistent sleep patterns. This includes maintaining a regular sleep schedule, even on weekends, to synchronize the body's internal clock. By adhering to a routine, the body becomes accustomed to a predictable sleep-wake cycle, promoting better sleep quality over time.

Mindful Nutrition for Better Sleep:

The holistic approach extends to dietary choices, recognizing the impact of nutrition on sleep. Avoiding stimulants like caffeine close to bedtime and opting for sleep-promoting foods can contribute to a more relaxed state before sleep. Additionally, staying adequately hydrated supports overall well-being, influencing sleep quality.

Stress Reduction Techniques:

Stress and sleep are intricately connected, and holistic sleep hygiene addresses this relationship by incorporating stress reduction techniques. Mindfulness practices, meditation, and relaxation exercises can help calm the mind, creating a conducive mental environment for sleep.

Limiting Screen Time:

In the digital age, electronic devices play a significant role in our lives, but they can adversely affect sleep. Holistic Sleep Hygiene advocates for limiting screen time before bedtime, as the blue light emitted by screens can disrupt the body's production of melatonin, a hormone essential for sleep.

Physical Activity as a Sleep Enhancer:

Regular physical activity is a cornerstone of holistic sleep hygiene. Engaging in moderate exercise not only contributes to overall health but also promotes better sleep. However, the timing of exercise is crucial, with intense workouts ideally scheduled earlier in the day.

Incorporating Relaxation Rituals:

Holistic sleep hygiene encourages the incorporation of relaxation rituals into the pre-sleep routine. This might involve activities such as reading a calming book, taking a warm bath, or practicing gentle stretches. These rituals signal the body that it's time to wind down, easing the transition into a restful night's sleep.

In essence, Holistic Sleep Hygiene is a comprehensive and integrative approach to sleep that acknowledges the intricate interplay of various factors. By addressing physical, mental, and environmental aspects, individuals can create a holistic sleep strategy tailored to their unique needs. Through conscious choices and mindful practices, the path to restorative and rejuvenating sleep becomes not just a goal but a sustainable and rewarding journey toward overall well-being.

The importance of sleep in holistic health

Quality sleep is a cornerstone of holistic health, playing a profound role in our overall well-being. In a fast-paced world where demands on our time and attention are ever-present, the importance of prioritizing sufficient and restorative sleep cannot be overstated. This critical aspect of our lives affects not just our physical health but also our mental and emotional states.

Body Restoration:

Sleep is a vital period during which our bodies undergo essential processes of repair and restoration. It is a time when tissues are healed, muscles are repaired, and the immune system is strengthened. The release of growth hormone occurs primarily during deep sleep, contributing to cellular regeneration and overall physical recovery. Chronic sleep deprivation, on the other hand, has been linked to increased susceptibility to illnesses, impaired immune function, and a higher risk of chronic conditions.

Cognitive Function:

A well-rested mind is a sharp mind. Sleep is intricately connected to cognitive functions such as memory consolidation, problem-solving abilities, and overall mental clarity. During the various stages of sleep, the brain processes information, forms connections, and consolidates memories, contributing to improved learning and better decision-making.

Emotional Well-being:

Insufficient sleep can significantly impact emotional well-being. It is associated with an increased likelihood of mood swings, irritability, and heightened emotional reactivity. On the contrary, adequate sleep fosters emotional resilience, better stress management, and an improved ability to navigate the challenges of daily life.

Hormonal Balance:

Sleep plays a crucial role in maintaining hormonal balance. Disruptions in sleep patterns can affect hormones related to hunger and satiety, potentially leading to weight gain and metabolic imbalances. Additionally, adequate sleep contributes to the regulation of stress hormones, promoting a healthier response to stressors in our environment.

Cardiovascular Health:

Holistic health encompasses the well-being of the entire cardiovascular system, and sleep plays a vital role in this regard. Sleep duration and quality have been linked to blood pressure regulation, inflammation levels, and overall cardiovascular health. Chronic sleep deprivation may contribute to an increased risk of heart disease and other cardiovascular issues.

Enhanced Physical Performance:

For those engaged in physical activities or sports, the importance of sleep cannot be emphasized enough. Athletes, in particular, benefit from optimal sleep for muscle recovery, coordination, and overall performance. Lack of sleep can lead to decreased endurance, slower recovery times, and increased susceptibility to injuries.

Longevity and Quality of Life:

Research consistently suggests a correlation between sufficient sleep and increased life expectancy. Quality sleep contributes to a healthier lifestyle, reduced risk of chronic diseases, and an overall improvement in the quality of life. It is a foundational element for achieving longevity and enjoying the various aspects of life to the fullest.

In conclusion, the importance of sleep in holistic health cannot be overstated. It is a time of restoration for the body, a rejuvenation of the mind, and an essential component of emotional and physical well-being. Prioritizing and nurturing healthy sleep patterns is an investment in one's overall health and vitality, contributing to a more vibrant, resilient, and fulfilling life.

Prioritizing restful sleep for optimal physical and mental functioning

prioritizing adequate and rejuvenating sleep is not merely a luxury; it's a cornerstone for optimal physical and mental functioning.

Physical Well-being:

Sleep is an indispensable component of our overall physical health. It is during sleep that our bodies undergo essential processes of repair and regeneration. Muscles heal, tissues rejuvenate, and the immune system strengthens. Chronic sleep deprivation, on the other hand, has been linked to a myriad of health issues, including an increased risk of cardiovascular diseases, compromised immune function, and hormonal imbalances.

Furthermore, prioritizing restful sleep contributes significantly to weight management. The intricate interplay of hormones responsible for appetite regulation is finely tuned during sleep. Lack of sleep disrupts this delicate balance, often leading to increased cravings for unhealthy foods and, consequently, weight gain.

Cognitive Functions:

A well-rested mind is a sharp mind. The cognitive benefits of prioritizing restful sleep are manifold. Memory consolidation, a process crucial for learning and retaining information, predominantly occurs during deep sleep phases. Additionally, adequate sleep enhances problem-solving skills, creativity, and overall cognitive performance.

Conversely, insufficient sleep impairs concentration, decision-making abilities, and emotional regulation. It fosters a state of mental fatigue that not only affects work productivity but also influences interpersonal relationships. Chronic sleep deprivation is associated with an increased risk of developing neurodegenerative conditions and mental health disorders, underlining the profound impact of sleep on the brain.

Emotional Resilience:

Prioritizing restful sleep is a cornerstone of emotional well-being. The emotional centers of the brain, intricately connected to the quality of sleep, depend on sufficient rest to function optimally. Adequate sleep fosters emotional resilience, enabling individuals to navigate stress, anxiety, and life's challenges more effectively.

Conversely, insufficient sleep heightens emotional reactivity. It can lead to increased irritability, heightened stress responses, and a reduced ability to cope with everyday pressures. Over time, chronic sleep deprivation contributes to the development or exacerbation of mood disorders, such as depression and anxiety.

Strategies for Prioritizing Restful Sleep:

1. **Consistent Sleep Schedule:**
   - Establish a regular sleep schedule by going to bed and waking up at the same time each day, even on weekends.
2. **Create a Relaxing Bedtime Routine:**

- Engage in calming activities before bedtime, such as reading a book, practicing relaxation exercises, or taking a warm bath.

3. **Optimize Sleep Environment:**

   - Ensure your sleep environment is conducive to rest – a comfortable mattress, dark curtains, and a cool room temperature can make a significant difference.

4. **Limit Stimulants:**

   - Reduce or eliminate stimulants like caffeine and nicotine in the hours leading up to bedtime.

5. **Digital Detox:**

   - Avoid electronic devices at least an hour before bedtime, as the blue light emitted can disrupt the production of the sleep-inducing hormone melatonin.

6. **Mindfulness and Relaxation Techniques:**

- Incorporate mindfulness meditation or deep breathing exercises to calm the mind and prepare it for rest.

In the relentless pursuit of productivity and success, the importance of prioritizing restful sleep should not be underestimated. It is not a passive indulgence but an active investment in one's physical and mental well-being. As we weave the fabric of our lives, let restful sleep be the thread that ensures resilience, vitality, and a foundation for the optimal functioning of both body and mind.

CHAPTER TEN:

Emotional Intelligence and Well-Being

Understanding Emotional Intelligence:

At its essence, emotional intelligence involves perceiving, understanding, managing, and using emotions to guide thoughts and actions. It encompasses self-awareness, recognizing one's emotions and their impact. Self-regulation is the ability to manage and control those emotions effectively, fostering resilience and adaptability.

Empathy and Social Skills:

Crucial components of emotional intelligence

include empathy, the capacity to comprehend and share the feelings of others. This ability to connect on an emotional level forms the foundation for positive social interactions. Coupled with adept social skills, emotional intelligence enhances communication, conflict resolution, and collaboration, enriching relationships both personally and professionally.

Emotional Intelligence and Well-Being:

Emotional intelligence and well-being are deeply intertwined. Individuals with high emotional intelligence tend to navigate stress, challenges, and conflicts more effectively. The ability to regulate emotions contributes to mental resilience, reducing the detrimental impact of stressors on mental health.

Moreover, heightened self-awareness allows for a more accurate understanding of personal needs and desires, fostering a sense of fulfillment and purpose.

Enhancing Mental Health:

In the realm of mental health, emotional intelligence serves as a powerful ally. Understanding one's emotions and those of others aids in the identification and management of mental health concerns. This self-awareness can be a crucial first step in seeking support or implementing strategies for coping with conditions such as anxiety or depression.

Professional Success and Leadership:

In the professional sphere, emotional intelligence is often a distinguishing factor between competent leaders and exceptional leaders. The ability to understand and connect with team members fosters a positive work environment. Leaders with high emotional intelligence can navigate complex interpersonal dynamics, resolve conflicts, and inspire their teams, contributing to overall workplace well-being.

Cultivating Emotional Intelligence:

Emotional intelligence is not fixed; it can be cultivated and refined over time. Practices such as mindfulness, self-reflection, and active listening contribute to the development of emotional intelligence. Engaging in meaningful conversations, seeking feedback, and embracing continuous learning are pathways toward honing these essential skills.

In the intricate dance of emotions, emotional intelligence emerges as the choreographer, orchestrating a symphony of well-being. From personal relationships to professional pursuits, its impact is profound. Cultivating emotional intelligence becomes a journey of self-discovery, a commitment to understanding the nuances of human emotions, and a conscious effort to foster a more compassionate and resilient existence. In embracing the principles of emotional intelligence, we unlock not only a deeper understanding of ourselves but also a pathway to a more fulfilling and harmonious life.

Understanding emotions and their role in holistic health

Emotions are the intricate threads that weave the fabric of our human experience. They are the visceral responses to the world around us, ranging from joy and love to sadness and anger. While often intangible, emotions play a profound role in shaping not only our mental well-being but also our physical health. In this exploration, we delve into the nuanced relationship between emotions and holistic health, recognizing the interconnected nature of mind, body, and spirit.

At the core of understanding emotions is the acknowledgment that they are not isolated events but rather dynamic forces that influence our entire being. Emotions are not confined to the mind alone; they have a tangible impact on physiological processes, shaping our health in ways that extend far beyond the realm of psychology.

Consider the physiological responses associated with different emotions. The elation of joy, for instance, triggers the release of endorphins, often referred to as "feel-good" hormones, which contribute to an overall sense of well-being. Conversely, experiences of chronic stress or unresolved emotions can manifest in physical symptoms – from elevated blood pressure to compromised immune function. This intricate interplay between emotions and the body underscores the importance of holistic health practices that address the complete spectrum of human experience.

Moreover, emotions serve as a barometer for our mental and spiritual health. They are messengers, offering insights into our inner landscape and alerting us to areas that may require attention and healing. A recurring sense of anxiety, for example, may prompt us to explore the root causes, guiding us towards therapeutic interventions or lifestyle adjustments that promote balance.

Holistic health, in essence, recognizes the inseparable connection between emotions, physical health, and overall well-being. It encourages an integrative approach that considers the emotional, mental, and spiritual dimensions alongside the physical. Practices such as mindfulness, meditation, and expressive therapies become invaluable tools in this holistic toolkit, offering individuals avenues to navigate, understand, and harmonize their emotional landscape.

In embracing holistic health, we embark on a journey towards self-discovery and self-care. It involves cultivating emotional intelligence – the ability to recognize, understand, and manage our own emotions, as well as empathize with the emotions of others. Through this process, we foster resilience, enhancing our capacity to navigate life's challenges with grace and equanimity.

Ultimately, understanding emotions in the context of holistic health invites us to view health not as the absence of disease but as a dynamic state of equilibrium encompassing physical vitality, mental clarity, emotional resilience, and spiritual well-being. It prompts us to embark on a holistic approach to health that honors the intricate dance between our thoughts, feelings, and bodily responses – a dance that, when harmonized, leads to a more vibrant and fulfilling life.

Developing emotional intelligence, coping mechanisms, and resilience

In the intricate tapestry of human experience, developing emotional intelligence stands as a beacon guiding us through the twists and turns of life. It is a journey that extends beyond mere self-awareness, transcending into a profound understanding and management of emotions, and ultimately, the cultivation of coping mechanisms and resilience.

Emotional Intelligence: The Foundation of Personal Growth

At its core, emotional intelligence encompasses the ability to recognize, understand, and manage one's own emotions, while also navigating and influencing the emotions of others. This journey commences with self-awareness, as individuals learn to identify and comprehend their emotional states. This heightened self-awareness lays the groundwork for emotional regulation, empowering individuals to manage their reactions in various situations.

Moreover, emotional intelligence extends to social awareness, allowing individuals to empathize with the feelings of others. By fostering empathetic connections, one not only builds healthier relationships but also contributes to a more harmonious community.

Cultivating Coping Mechanisms: A Vital Skill Set

Life, with its kaleidoscope of experiences, is bound to present challenges. Developing emotional intelligence involves equipping oneself with effective coping mechanisms to navigate these challenges with grace and resilience. Coping mechanisms serve as the tools in our emotional toolkit, enabling us to respond to stressors, setbacks, and adversities in a healthy and constructive manner.

Whether it's through mindfulness practices, engaging in hobbies, or seeking support from others, the art of coping involves finding adaptive strategies that resonate with individual needs. This journey towards effective coping is about transforming challenges into opportunities for personal growth, fostering a mindset that sees resilience not as a reaction but as a proactive response to life's complexities.

Resilience: Flourishing Amidst Adversity

Resilience is the cornerstone of emotional intelligence, representing the capacity to bounce back from setbacks and emerge stronger. It's not about avoiding challenges but facing them with an unwavering spirit. Resilience involves cultivating a mindset that perceives setbacks as temporary and views failures as stepping stones toward success.

Building resilience entails embracing change, adapting to unforeseen circumstances, and maintaining a positive outlook even in the face of adversity. By acknowledging that setbacks are an integral part of life, individuals can harness their emotional intelligence to navigate challenges, learn from experiences, and emerge with newfound strength and wisdom.

In conclusion, the journey of developing emotional intelligence, coping mechanisms, and resilience is a dynamic and lifelong process. It's about understanding the intricacies of human emotions, equipping oneself with adaptive tools to navigate life's challenges, and fostering a spirit that not only withstands adversity but flourishes in its wake. As we embark on this journey, let us embrace the richness of our emotional landscape, fortify our coping mechanisms, and cultivate resilience as we navigate the ever-evolving tapestry of life.

Holistic Beauty and Self-Care

Holistic beauty and self-care represent an integrated approach to well-being that extends beyond traditional beauty practices. Holistic beauty emphasizes the interconnectedness of the mind, body, and spirit, recognizing that external beauty is a reflection of internal health. This approach promotes a comprehensive and balanced lifestyle that nurtures physical, mental, and emotional health.

In holistic beauty, skincare is not just about external treatments but also involves nourishing the body from within. A focus on a nutritious diet, hydration, and mindful eating plays a crucial role. Incorporating antioxidant-rich foods, vitamins, and minerals contributes to skin health and radiance. Additionally, staying hydrated supports overall bodily functions, including skin hydration.

Holistic self-care encompasses practices that go beyond surface-level relaxation. Meditation, mindfulness, and stress management techniques are key components. These practices not only benefit mental well-being but also contribute to a healthy complexion, as stress can impact skin health.

Physical activity is another integral aspect of holistic self-care. Regular exercise not only enhances circulation and promotes a healthy weight but also releases endorphins, contributing to a positive mood. Yoga, in particular, is often embraced in holistic beauty routines for its combination of physical movement, breathwork, and mental focus.

Choosing natural and non-toxic beauty products aligns with holistic beauty principles. Many holistic enthusiasts prioritize products with minimal chemicals and opt for organic or cruelty-free options. This approach is not only about achieving external beauty but also supporting overall health and environmental sustainability.

Holistic self-care extends to sleep hygiene as well. Quality sleep is essential for cellular repair, and lack of it can lead to skin issues. Establishing a consistent sleep routine and creating a calming bedtime environment contribute to both physical and mental well-being.

A holistic approach also emphasizes the importance of self-love and acceptance. Fostering a positive self-image and practicing self-compassion are crucial aspects of holistic beauty. This involves appreciating oneself beyond physical appearance and embracing individual uniqueness.

In summary, holistic beauty and self-care represent a comprehensive lifestyle approach that acknowledges the interconnectedness of physical, mental, and emotional well-being. By integrating practices that nurture the mind, body, and spirit, individuals can cultivate a radiant and balanced sense of beauty that goes beyond the superficial.

Holistic beauty and self-care encompass a comprehensive approach to well-being, emphasizing the interconnectedness of physical, mental, and emotional aspects of an individual's health. It goes beyond superficial aesthetics, promoting a balance that radiates from within. Keynotes for readers to consider:

1. **Mind-Body Connection:**

    o   Holistic beauty emphasizes the inseparable link between mental and physical health.

    o   Practices like meditation, mindfulness, and deep breathing contribute to a positive mindset, reflecting in one's appearance.

2. **Nutrition and Nourishment:**

    o   A holistic approach to beauty involves mindful eating, focusing on nutrient-dense foods that support overall health.

    o   Hydrating adequately and incorporating antioxidants in the diet can enhance skin vitality.

3. **Natural and Sustainable Beauty:**

    o   Holistic beauty encourages the use of clean, eco-friendly beauty products.

- Sustainable choices reduce environmental impact, aligning with a broader sense of well-being.

4. **Stress Management:**

   - Chronic stress can adversely affect both physical and mental health.
   - Incorporating stress-relieving practices like yoga, journaling, or spending time in nature is essential for holistic self-care.

5. **Quality Sleep:**

   - Prioritizing sufficient and quality sleep is integral to holistic beauty.
   - Sleep supports cellular repair, contributes to a healthy complexion, and enhances overall vitality.

6. **Movement and Exercise:**

- Regular physical activity boosts circulation, promoting a healthy glow.
- Holistic self-care includes finding joy in movement, whether through yoga, dance, or other forms of exercise.

7. **Self-Reflection and Emotional Wellness:**

- Understanding and addressing emotional well-being is crucial for holistic beauty.
- Practices like therapy, self-reflection, and cultivating positive relationships contribute to a balanced emotional state.

8. **Individualized Beauty Routines:**

- Recognizing that each person's beauty needs are unique is fundamental in holistic beauty.

- Tailoring skincare and self-care routines to individual preferences and skin types promotes personalized well-being.

9. **Connection to Nature:**

- Spending time outdoors fosters a sense of connection to nature, promoting holistic balance.
- Natural elements can inspire mindfulness and a sense of tranquility.

10. **Gratitude and Positivity:**

- Holistic beauty involves cultivating gratitude and maintaining a positive outlook.
- Expressing gratitude and focusing on positive aspects of life contribute to a radiant aura.

In embracing holistic beauty and self-care, readers are encouraged to adopt an integrative mindset, recognizing that true beauty emanates from a harmonious balance of physical, mental, and emotional health

Integrating natural beauty practices, mindful grooming, and self-love

Integrating Natural Beauty Practices, Mindful Grooming, and Self-Love" is a holistic guide that delves into the intricate relationship between self-care, natural beauty practices, and fostering a deep sense of self-love. The narrative unfolds through a comprehensive exploration of the interconnected elements that contribute to a harmonious and healthy embodiment of one's true self.

Keynotes for Readers:

Holistic Wellness Approach:

1. Emphasizing a holistic approach, the guide advocates for the integration of physical, mental, and emotional well-being. By aligning natural beauty practices with mindful grooming routines, readers are guided towards a more complete and sustainable sense of wellness.

Embracing Natural Beauty:

2. The narrative celebrates individuality and encourages readers to embrace their natural beauty. From skincare routines rooted in organic ingredients to appreciating unique physical attributes, the guide fosters a positive

self-image by highlighting the beauty in authenticity.

Mindful Grooming Rituals:

3. The guide introduces readers to the transformative power of mindful grooming rituals. It explores the significance of intentional self-care, encouraging readers to view grooming not just as a routine but as a meditative practice that nurtures the mind, body, and spirit.

Cultural and Historical Perspectives:

4. Providing a rich tapestry of cultural and historical perspectives, the guide traces the evolution of beauty practices. By

understanding the diverse roots of self-care traditions, readers gain a deeper appreciation for the rituals they incorporate into their own lives.

Sustainable Practices:

5. A key focus lies in promoting sustainability. The guide encourages eco-friendly choices in beauty and grooming, fostering a sense of responsibility towards the environment. This includes exploring cruelty-free products, reducing waste, and adopting practices that contribute positively to the planet.

Self-Love Journey:

6. At the core of the narrative is the transformative journey towards self-love. Through reflective exercises, affirmations, and practical tips, readers are guided in developing a profound connection with themselves. This self-love journey becomes the foundation for a positive and fulfilling life.

Empowerment Through Knowledge:

7. The guide empowers readers by providing in-depth knowledge about skincare, grooming techniques, and the science behind beauty practices. Armed with this understanding, individuals can make informed choices that align with

their values and contribute to their overall well-being.

Connection to Mental Health:

8. Recognizing the inseparable link between physical appearance and mental health, the guide addresses the importance of self-compassion and self-care in cultivating a resilient mindset. It encourages readers to view beauty practices as tools for enhancing mental well-being.

In essence, "Body" serves as a comprehensive roadmap for readers seeking a profound and transformative journey towards embracing their natural beauty, cultivating mindful grooming practices, and fostering a deep sense of self-love that radiates from within. Integrating Natural Beauty Practices, Mindful Grooming, and Self-Love"

In the pursuit of holistic well-being, the essence of caring for one's body extends beyond mere aesthetics, delving into the realms of natural beauty practices, mindful grooming, and self-love. This comprehensive exploration embraces a harmonious approach to body care, resonating with readers seeking a deeper connection with their physical selves.

Natural beauty practices form the cornerstone of this journey, emphasizing the use of organic, cruelty-free products and embracing the inherent beauty that comes from nurturing the body in its most authentic state. From nourishing skincare routines to embracing one's natural hair texture, the narrative encourages readers to celebrate their unique features, fostering a sense of self-appreciation rooted in authenticity.

Mindful grooming becomes a pivotal aspect, transcending routine into a conscious ritual. The focus shifts from mere maintenance to an intentional, meditative experience, where each act of grooming becomes an opportunity for self-reflection and self-expression. This approach fosters a heightened awareness of the body's needs and cultivates a mindful connection to the present moment, the empowerment derived from understanding that self-love is not a destination but a continuous journey. The narrative unfolds as a guide, urging individuals to cultivate self-love by embracing their bodies at every stage, acknowledging imperfections as unique marks of their personal journey. Readers are encouraged to shed societal standards and embrace a positive self-image, fostering resilience against external pressures.

The integration of natural beauty practices, mindful grooming, and self-love is not a mere aesthetic pursuit but a transformative experience that transcends physical appearances. It becomes a holistic approach to well-being, where the body becomes a canvas for self-expression, and self-love becomes the driving force behind every action. This narrative serves as an empowering manifesto, inspiring readers to embark on a journey of self-discovery, embracing their bodies as vessels of strength, beauty, and authenticity.

How to Sustaining Holistic Health Practices

Sustaining holistic health practices involves adopting a comprehensive approach to well-being that encompasses physical, mental, and emotional dimensions. This holistic approach recognizes the interconnectedness of various aspects of health, emphasizing the importance of balance and harmony. Here are some keynotes to guide readers in embracing and sustaining holistic health practices:

1. **Mind-Body Connection:**
   - Acknowledge the profound link between mental and physical health.

- Embrace practices like mindfulness, meditation, and yoga to foster a strong mind-body connection.

2. **Nutrition as Nourishment:**
   - Prioritize whole, nutrient-dense foods to support overall health.
   - Understand the significance of a well-balanced diet in providing essential nutrients for optimal bodily functions.

3. **Physical Activity and Exercise:**
   - Engage in regular physical activity that aligns with personal preferences and goals.
   - Recognize the diverse benefits of exercise, from cardiovascular health to stress reduction.

4. **Emotional Well-being:**

- Cultivate emotional intelligence and self-awareness.
- Establish healthy coping mechanisms for stress, such as journaling, art, or connecting with loved ones.

5. **Quality Sleep:**
   - Prioritize sufficient and quality sleep as a foundation for overall well-being.
   - Establish a consistent sleep routine and create a conducive sleep environment.

6. **Holistic Healthcare Practices:**
   - Explore alternative and complementary therapies like acupuncture, chiropractic care, or herbal medicine.
   - Integrate holistic approaches alongside conventional medical

care for a well-rounded health strategy.

7. **Environmental Awareness:**
   - Understand the impact of the environment on health.
   - Foster eco-friendly habits to promote a sustainable and health-conscious lifestyle.

8. **Community and Social Connections:**
   - Recognize the importance of social relationships for mental and emotional health.
   - Build and maintain strong social connections to create a supportive community.

9. **Stress Management:**
   - Develop effective stress management techniques, such as deep breathing exercises or time management strategies.

- Prioritize activities that promote relaxation and rejuvenation.

10. **Continuous Learning and Growth:**
    - Embrace a growth mindset and engage in lifelong learning.
    - Stay curious and open-minded, exploring new ways to enhance personal development.

11. **Self-Care Rituals:**
    - Establish regular self-care practices that align with individual preferences.
    - Prioritize self-reflection and ensure personal needs are met to sustain long-term well-being.

12. **Holistic Goal Setting:**
    - Set holistic goals that encompass physical, mental, and emotional aspects.

- Break down goals into manageable steps to create a sense of achievement and motivation.

In sustaining holistic health practices, individuals are encouraged to view health as a dynamic and interconnected journey, recognizing that small, consistent efforts across various dimensions contribute to overall well-being.

Encouraging readers to embrace holistic health as an ongoing journey for a fulfilling life

Embracing holistic health is not merely a destination but a transformative journey that encompasses the integration of physical, mental, and emotional well-being. It goes beyond conventional approaches, encouraging readers to adopt a comprehensive and sustainable lifestyle that nurtures every facet of their existence.

At its core, holistic health recognizes the intricate interconnectedness of various aspects of life. Physically, it involves nourishing the body through balanced nutrition, regular exercise, and adequate sleep. Mental well-being is cultivated through practices like mindfulness, meditation, and stress management, fostering a harmonious relationship between the mind and body.

Embracing holistic health extends beyond the individual, encompassing interpersonal relationships and community connections.

Building and maintaining healthy relationships contribute significantly to one's overall well-being. Cultivating a supportive social network enhances emotional resilience and provides a foundation for personal growth.

The journey towards holistic health is dynamic, acknowledging that well-being is an ongoing process rather than a static achievement. It encourages readers to be proactive in self-care, making conscious choices that align with their values and contribute to a fulfilling life. This might involve exploring new hobbies, learning, and continuously seeking personal development opportunities.

A crucial element of holistic health is environmental consciousness. Recognizing the impact of our surroundings on well-being, it encourages sustainable practices that not only benefit individuals but also contribute to the well-being of the planet. This might include embracing eco-friendly habits, connecting with nature, and fostering a sense of environmental responsibility.

Moreover, holistic health is not a one-size-fits-all approach. It recognizes and respects individual differences, promoting a personalized journey tailored to one's unique needs and circumstances. Readers are encouraged to listen to their bodies, understand their emotional landscapes, and make choices that align with their authentic selves.

In essence, embracing holistic health as an ongoing journey is an invitation to live a life of purpose, balance, and fulfillment. It empowers individuals to take charge of their well-being, recognizing that true health encompasses not just the absence of illness but a vibrant and flourishing existence in all its dimensions.

Embarking on a journey toward holistic health is an empowering decision that encompasses the well-being of mind, body, and spirit. Picture this transformative expedition as a continuous path, not a destination; a perpetual evolution fostering a fulfilling and vibrant life.

Keynote 1: Mind-Body Connection

Unveil the profound interconnection between mental and physical health. Encourage readers to recognize that a harmonious mind-body relationship is pivotal for overall well-being. Embrace practices like mindfulness, meditation, and yoga to nurture this synergy.

Keynote 2: Nutrition as Fuel for Vitality

Highlight the significance of conscious eating choices. Fueling the body with nutrient-dense foods not only enhances physical health but also influences mental clarity and emotional stability. Encourage readers to view their diet as a source of vitality and energy.

Keynote 3: Cultivating Emotional Intelligence

Guide readers to explore and understand their emotions. Emotional intelligence is the compass that directs us through life's challenges. Encourage practices like journaling, therapy, or meditation to foster self-awareness and resilience.

Keynote 4: Physical Activity for Lifelong Wellness

Stress the importance of regular exercise, not solely for physical fitness but as a holistic approach to well-being. Engaging in activities that bring joy fosters a sustainable commitment to an active lifestyle, contributing to both mental and physical health.

Keynote 5: Balancing Work and Personal Life

Acknowledge the demands of daily life but emphasize the need for a balance that nurtures overall wellness. Encourage setting boundaries, practicing time management, and prioritizing self-care to prevent burnout and enhance life satisfaction.

Keynote 6: Nurturing Relationships

Highlight the impact of meaningful connections on holistic health. Encourage readers to cultivate positive relationships, invest time in loved ones, and establish healthy boundaries. A supportive social network is a cornerstone of a fulfilling life.

Keynote 7: Continuous Learning and Growth

Stress the significance of intellectual and personal development. Embracing a mindset of continual learning contributes to a sense of purpose and accomplishment. Encourage readers to explore new interests and challenge themselves regularly.

Keynote 8: Connecting with Nature

Remind readers of the therapeutic benefits of nature. Spending time outdoors, whether through walks, hikes, or simply immersing oneself in natural surroundings, can have a profound impact on mental and emotional well-being.

Keynote 9: Mindful Technology Use

Address the role of technology in our lives. Encourage readers to adopt mindful practices regarding screen time and social media usage.

Promote a healthy digital balance that allows for genuine connections and reduces stress.

Keynote 10: Gratitude as a Daily Practice

Instill the habit of gratitude into daily life. A grateful mindset fosters positivity, resilience, and an appreciation for life's journey. Encourage readers to reflect on the positives, no matter how small, and incorporate gratitude into their routine.

By embracing holistic health as an ongoing journey, readers can create a fulfilling and vibrant life, where each component works in harmony to cultivate a sense of purpose, resilience, and joy.

www.ingramcontent.com/pod-product-compliance
Lightning Source LLC
Chambersburg PA
CBHW080925260726
48661CB00010B/3804